Almost everyone, at some tim
with the problem of cor
appropriate method of birth
suits the lifestyle of the user –
book will help couples to ma

In particular this book conc
regulation – the intrauterine
different IUD models which are available are described, and the procedures entailed in having an IUD fitted are explained. Many of the common questions which women ask about IUDs are answered; How effective is the IUD? How safe is it? Are there any side effects to its use?

Robert Snowden, who is co-ordinator of the UK IUD Research Network, uses research data which has been collected over a period of 15 years to answer these questions and to explain the likelihood of the occurrence of side effects which different women might experience. The IUD does not necessarily suit every woman, nor is the IUD the most appropriate method of birth control to use at all stages of a woman's reproductive life. Women, and their medical advisors, will find this book a valuable source of information which will help them to make a wise decision in their choice of contraceptive method.

Also by Robert Snowden,
and published by Allen and Unwin Publishers

with Elizabeth Snowden
The Gift of a Child

with Elizabeth Snowden and Duncan Mitchell
Artificial Reproduction: A Social Investigation

with Duncan Mitchell
The Artificial Family: A Consideration of Artificial Insemination by Donor

THE I.U.D.

A WOMAN'S GUIDE

Recommended by the Family Planning Association

Dr Robert Snowden

London
UNWIN PAPERBACKS
Boston Sydney

First published in Great Britain by Unwin Paperbacks 1986

UNWIN ® PAPERBACKS
40 Museum Street, London WC1A 1LU, UK

Unwin Paperbacks
Park Lane, Hemel Hempstead, Herts HP2 4TE, UK

Allen & Unwin Australia Pty Ltd
8 Napier Street, North Sydney, NSW 2060, Australia

Unwin Paperbacks with the
Port Nicholson Press
PO Box 11-838 Wellington, New Zealand

British Library Cataloguing in Publication Data

Snowden, Robert
The IUD : a woman's guide.
1. Intrauterine contraceptives
I. Title
613.9'435 RG137.3

ISBN 0–04–612037–8

Printed in Great Britain by Hazell, Watson & Viney Limited
Member of the BPCC Group, Aylesbury, Bucks.

CONTENTS

Line illustrations by Maggie Raynor, apart from Figure 1c by Laura McKechnie.

ACKNOWLEDGEMENTS

Since research into the use of intrauterine devices (IUDs) was started in 1968, over 40,000 individual IUD users have contributed to the information on which this book is based. The medical teams in each of the forty-six family planning clinics who cooperate in the UK IUD Research Network spend many hours, without remuneration, completing research forms and answering enquiries about the IUD service they provide. These two groups are joined by the research team at the Institute of Population Studies, University of Exeter, which prepares, computes and assists in the writing of research reports. My sincere thanks go to them all.

Special thanks go to Dr Margaret Jackson who has taught me so much about IUDs over the years and to Dr Elizabeth (Libby) Wilson who helped with Chapter 4 *Having an IUD fitted.* The IUD Research Network was set up in 1971 and still exists mainly because of the continuing enthusiasm of the twenty-three doctors who act as the principal investigators responsible for collecting the information about IUDs in the participating family planning clinics. I have listed these dedicated professionals below.

Whilst personally accepting any shortcomings in this book, its existence owes much to the work, advice and support of these colleagues.

Principal investigators in the UK IUD Research Network

E. Andrews *(Taunton)*
J. Bland *(Nuneaton)*
E. J. Burton *(Barnsley)*

G. C. Cardy *(Wiltshire)*
J. D. Clark *(Plymouth)*
M. L. Cox *(Nuneaton)*
J. Dewsbury *(Birmingham)*
A. Foxell *(Guildford)*
E. Gregson *Consultant*
B. Hanson *(Wiltshire)*
M. C. N. Jackson *Consultant*
J. P. Lawson *(London-Hammersmith)*
R. Lincoln *(Norwich)*
M. Lloyd *(Exeter)*
A. Main *(London-Richmond)*
E. Mayall *(Exeter)*
J. North *(Southampton)*
S. Richardson *(West Yorkshire)*
R. Snowden *(Co-ordinator)*
J. Tattersall *(Sheffield)*
A. Thomas *(Newport)*
E. M. Watt *(Bristol)*
E. Wilson *(Glasgow)*
E. Wishart *(Birmingham)*

FOREWORD

by Dr Mike Smith

The IUD – Intra-Uterine Device – is the chosen contraceptive for up to a million British women. On behalf of them, and many millions more in the rest of the world, I welcome Dr Robert Snowden's fact-packed and readable book.

Based, as it is, on detailed and extensive research work plus Dr Snowden's experience spread over two decades, *The IUD: A Woman's Guide* provides all of us with the kind of insights that we have come to expect from him – and all of us includes not only the women to whom the book is primarily directed, but also those who 'fit' IUD's, run surgeries and clinics, or are just interested in the IUD and how it works. Dr Snowden has not let us down. Once again, with this book, he has enhanced his international reputation as the leading expert in this field.

It is likely that the reader who will benefit most from this book will be the IUD user (or wearer), or potential user herself. From Dr Snowden's general advice about the IUD and why it may be the best method for you in particular, there is detail enough for the most discriminating reader, who may have doubts about using it at all.

As with all forms of contraception, that's how it should be. If you decide after reading this book and before going to your doctor for advice that the IUD seems to be what you need – your doctor should be delighted, knowing that an informed contraceptive user is the one who will be most satisfied, and so continue, with the method chosen. Dr Snowden has, and justifiably so, told us this often enough over the years. His research has also told us that the properly informed woman using an IUD is the one who is the least likely to suffer any side-effects – and that includes the small but known risk of pregnancy.

What more is there to say but that I thoroughly recommend Dr Snowden's *The IUD: A Woman's Guide* to you.

Dr Mike Smith

INTRODUCTION

The first task is to reach some agreement about what a device which is placed in a woman's uterus for the purpose of preventing a pregnancy is to be called. Some people refer to it as the 'coil', others the 'loop' and those who pretend to greater knowledge of the subject argue – sometimes heatedly – over whether it should be called an IUD or an IUCD. Most medical practitioners in the United Kingdom prefer to use the term IUCD or 'Intrauterine Contraceptive Device', whereas the international convention has been to use the abbreviation IUD for 'Intrauterine Device'. The World Health Organisation (WHO) debated this issue in 1967 voted for the international version but, nevertheless, most members of the medical profession in the UK continue to use the abbreviation IUCD. As a great deal of the research in which I have been engaged has been international in scope, I am used to the term 'IUD' and so have opted to use it throughout this book.

Having decided what these devices are to be called, I must confess to some hesitation about my qualifications for writing about them. A book for women who are contemplating or experiencing IUD use, which is written by a man who has neither used an IUD nor ever fitted one may need some explanation. I first began collecting information about IUDs in 1966. This began quite by accident, and was mainly due to a need to earn some money to help keep a wife and three daughters whilst taking a psychology degree as a 'mature' student. I began working in the Exeter Family Planning Clinic with Dr Margaret Jackson, a family planning pioneer, who started many clinics in the South West of England at a time when family planning was not openly discussed as it is today. This outstanding doctor opened the Exeter clinic in 1930, fitted her first IUD in 1939 and retired fifty-two years later in 1982, during which time she helped many thousands of women. From these beginnings the collection and interpretation of information about IUDs has steadily grown. This work now extends to forty-six family planning clinics situated in different parts of the UK staffed by teams of doctors, nurses and assistants who cooperate in an organisation called the UK IUD Research Network. This research is noteworthy in two important respects: first, it takes as its starting point the individual woman's view of the IUD as a method of contraception; second, the doctors who cooperate together in these research activities do so without personal remuneration. When this work started, the effects of intrauterine contraception had not been closely studied in the UK. Also there was no identification of the different types of IUD model when assessing them in terms of their ability to prevent a pregnancy; an IUD was an IUD and that was that!

In twenty years of research, the UK IUD Research Network has studied in excess of a dozen IUD models and has been asked to comment on numerous newly invented devices which never made it into commercial production. In the early days it seemed that every meeting I attended to talk about IUD research included a conversation with someone who had developed – or, more correctly, was in the process of developing – a new IUD model which could be of benefit to so many women if only it could be effectively marketed. These people were mostly gynaecologists and always men. In all these twenty years I have never come across an IUD that has been invented by a woman! The reason for this proliferation of IUD models may partly be explained by the absence of an agreed and consistent body of knowledge about IUD design. New IUDs were invented in an idiosyncratic way and tended to follow fads and fashions in design rather than any scientific design principles. More recently regulations for the production and manufacture of new devices have been introduced, and rigorous standards must be met in the testing of new devices before they are made available for general use.

But perhaps even more important than the IUD inventors have been the staff who fit the IUDs at the clinics and the women who have dealt patiently with the repeated questioning about their experiences of using IUDs over the years. As a result of all the information that has been collected, and the research findings that have been presented, there is one feature of IUD provision that stands out: if intrauterine contraception is to be used satisfactorily, the inter-relationship between the type of IUD, the individual requirements of the woman being fitted, and the skill and care of the doctor is of the utmost importance. Each factor is crucial and to emphasise any one of them at the expense of the others would be a serious mistake.

Perhaps the most important change in attitudes over recent years is reflected by the fact that doctors now refer to the 'fitting' of an IUD rather than to its 'insertion'. The distinction is important because 'fitting' implies meeting the needs of an individual woman who will wear an IUD over a period of time, whereas 'inserting' implies merely a technical procedure for putting an IUD into a uterus. To 'fit' an IUD implies that the individual needs and feelings of the whole woman are seen as being important rather than just the technicalities of her reproductive system. It also suggests that the service being provided starts with the needs of the person using the service and that all other considerations should be secondary to this.

I have been privileged to conduct research into the use of IUDs over many years. I hope the following pages, which have resulted from this research, will assist those women who are currently wearing an IUD or those who may be contemplating its use.

July 1985

R. Snowden, PhD
Institute of Population Studies,
University of Exeter

CHAPTER 1

Why choose an IUD?

An intrauterine device is a small object, usually made of plastic but sometimes made of other materials, which is carefully placed in a woman's womb or uterus for contraceptive purposes. The insertion of the device is not difficult, but as the size, shape and position of the uterus cannot be predicted precisely in advance, most IUDs are fitted by qualified doctors who have received specialist training.

Before being able to understand how IUDs work, how they are placed in the uterus, and the experience of women using these devices, some knowledge of the female reproductive system is required. For instance, when shown an IUD for the first time, many women are surprised to see how small it is. It is, of course, designed to 'fit' the 'typical' **uterus**. This is pear-shaped and, in the non-pregnant state, its internal measurements are about equivalent in size to the area created by placing together the tips of the thumb and middle finger of one hand. This small organ lies in the centre of the pelvis with the narrow part of the structure pointing downwards. The uterus is linked to the **vagina** by means of a narrow passage called the **cervical canal**. (See Figure 1a and b.) The opening of the cervical canal into the vagina is called the **external os** and the point where it enters the uterus, the **internal os.**

At the upper end of the uterus and at its widest point, there are two **fallopian tubes**, one on each side. These normally carry one **ovum** (or egg) at a time from the **ovary** to the uterus. If fertilisation of the ovum by a sperm takes place, it usually does so in the fallopian tube. When a fertilised ovum reaches the uterus it will embed itself in the **endometrium** or lining of the uterus. The endometrium becomes thickened in order to receive the developing ovum and to provide it with an adequate blood supply. However, if the ovum is not fertilised it will be shed from the uterus along with the thickened layers of endometrium (which are no longer needed) at the time of **menstruation**.

When viewed along a straight line down the middle of the body the uterus is usually in the centre of the pelvis but its position in terms of how close it lies to the front or back of the body is less easy to predict. The uterus does not always maintain a straight line; in many women it is bent towards the front of the body, though in others it leans towards the back. Roughly speaking, this gives three possible positions of the uterus: where it bends towards the front of the body it is known as an **anteverted uterus** (see Figure 2a); where it bends towards the back of the body it is called a **retroverted uterus** (see Figure 2b); and where it lies on a straight line between the two, it is described as being in the **mid-position** (see Figure 2c). Our own research has shown that approximately 70 per cent of women attending clinics for an IUD fitting have an anteverted uterus, 19 per cent a retroverted uterus and 11 per cent have a uterus in the

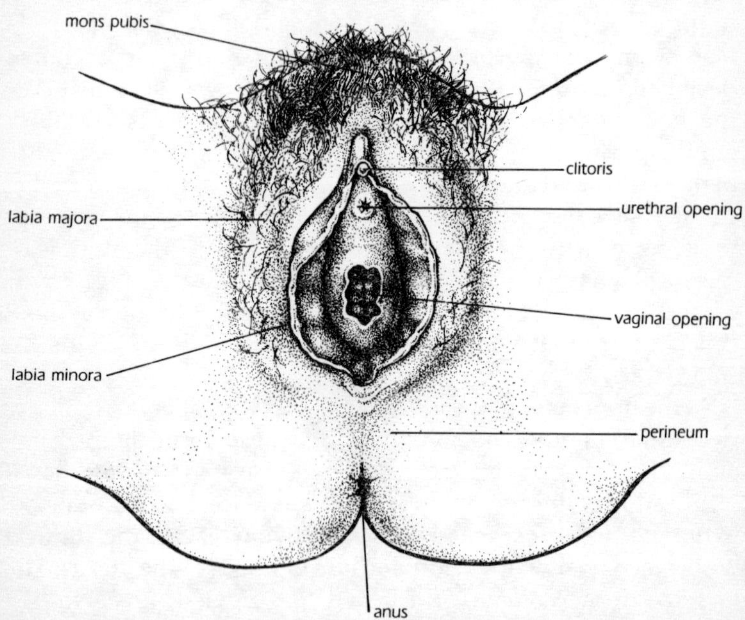

Figure 1a The female reproductive organs – front view

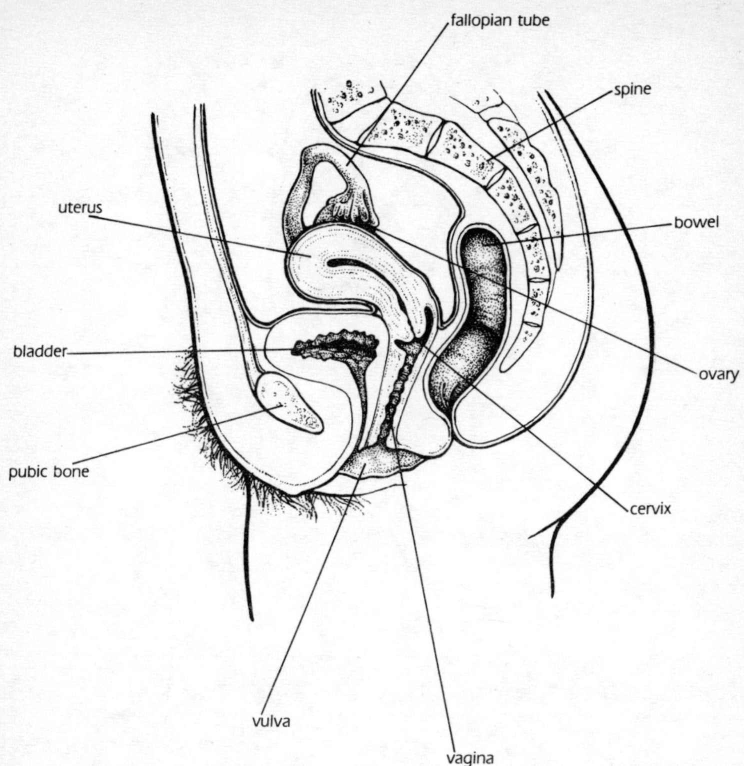

Figure 1b The female reproductive organs – cross section

mid-position. This knowledge is important because it explains why the doctor needs to do a manual pelvic examination immediately before fitting an IUD. The shape, size and direction of the uterus all contribute to determining whether or not an IUD should be fitted, and how best to fit an appropriate IUD with the minimum of discomfort.

This then is the basic information about the reproductive system required when considering the use of an intrauterine device as a method of contraception. Each of the terms used will come up again when specific aspects of IUD use are considered.

But what of the IUD itself? Put simply, the IUD has to perform five functions, all of which are dependent in some way on each other. It must:

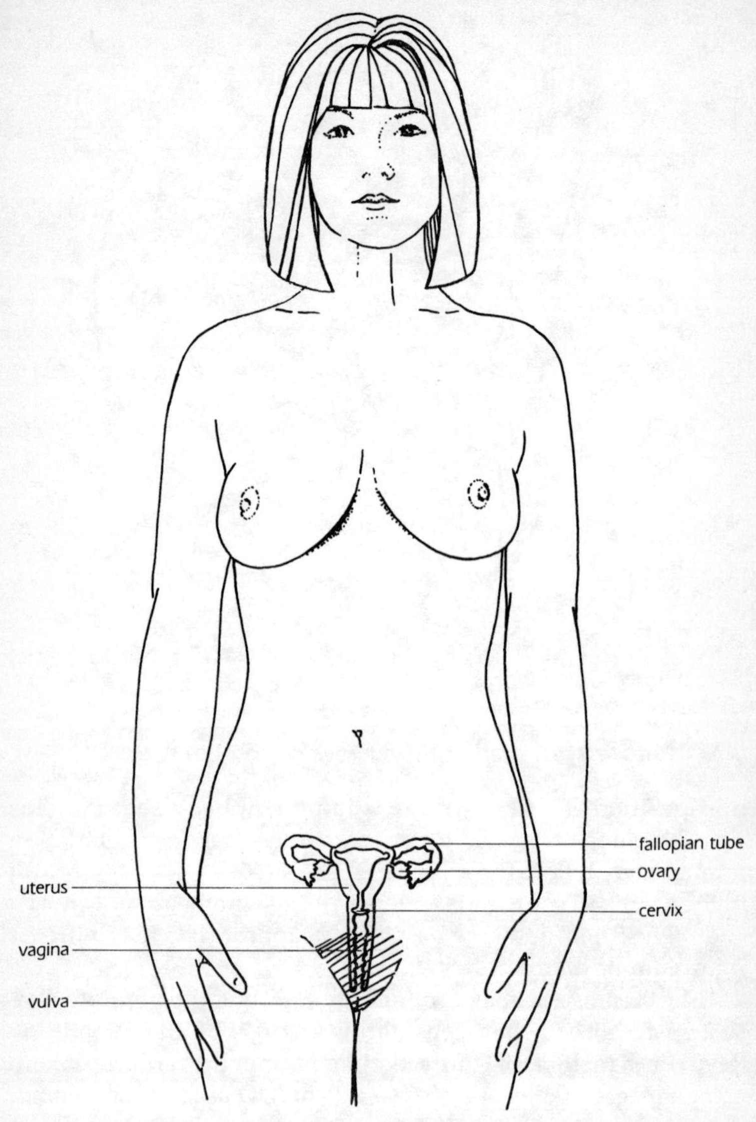

Figure 1c Position of the female reproductive organs

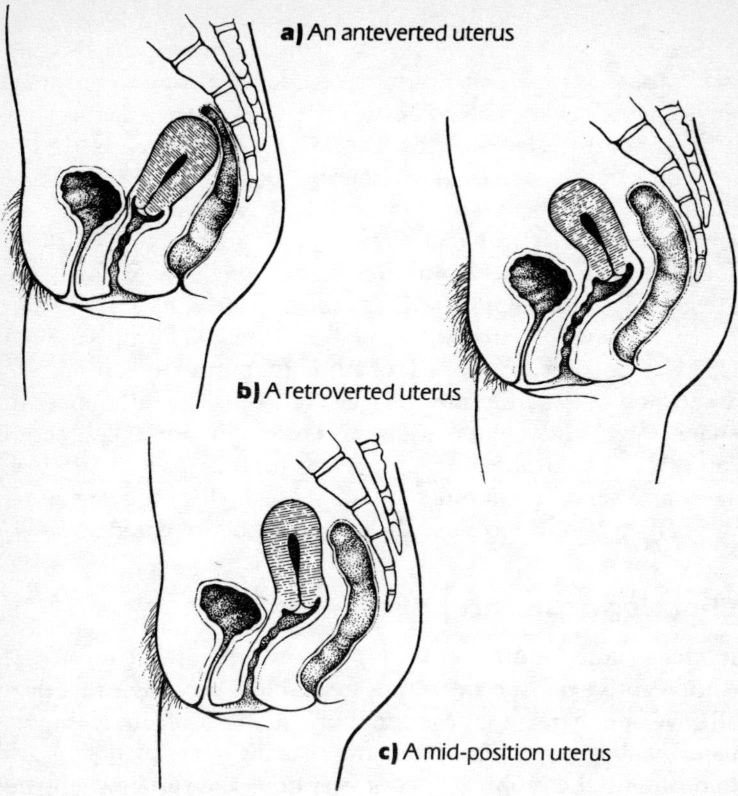

Figure 2 The three possible positions of the uterus

i) prevent an unwanted pregnancy
ii) be easy to insert into the uterus
iii) be easy to remove when this is desired
iv) avoid the causation of unwanted side effects
v) not interfere with a return to fertility once the IUD has been removed.

The development of IUDs in the last seventy-five years has been guided by the need to satisfy these five requirements, but it has met with only partial success. This partial rather than full success is due to the conflicting demands of the requirements themselves. An IUD that is easy to fit and easy to remove is more likely to be expelled from the uterus than one that is more difficult to fit and remove. A device which expels easily inevitably has a lower degree of protection against pregnancy. A device which is unlikely to be expelled from the uterus (because of its shape and size) is often associated with an increase in the unwanted side effects of discomfort or increased menstrual bleeding. It seems that if one problem is resolved, its resolution creates additional problems elsewhere. To get all five issues into some kind of balance continues to be a major task for those attempting to develop new IUD models.

The IUD models currently available in the UK, Europe and the USA have been developed bearing in mind the difficulties associated with earlier models (see Figure 3). The differences in shape, size and composition of these modern IUDs are a reflection of a number of attempts to learn from past experience. They also serve to remind us that the ideal IUD which meets all the demands of the consumer has still to be invented.

Choosing a contraceptive

It does not require detailed research knowledge of the contraceptive products currently available to recognise that they all have one characteristic in common – they are all unpleasant to use. But almost all of us, at sometime during our adult lives, have to deal with the problem of contraception. The very few who do not have this concern are those who, by choice or accident, are never likely to experience a sexual relationship with a member of the opposite sex. Even those couples who are in the unhappy position of being unable to have children but who have a normal and healthy sexual relationship, have usually experienced the use of contraception before their infertility was recognised. Conversation with such couples has revealed that despite their deep-seated hurt at not being able to have a child of their own, one positive feature is often recognised. To enjoy a hetero-sexual relationship in the absence of any concerns about contraception is a luxury – which they would doubtless rather do without if it meant being able to have a child of their own. But the joy of sex uninhibited by the thoughts of contraception is something most people can only dream of.

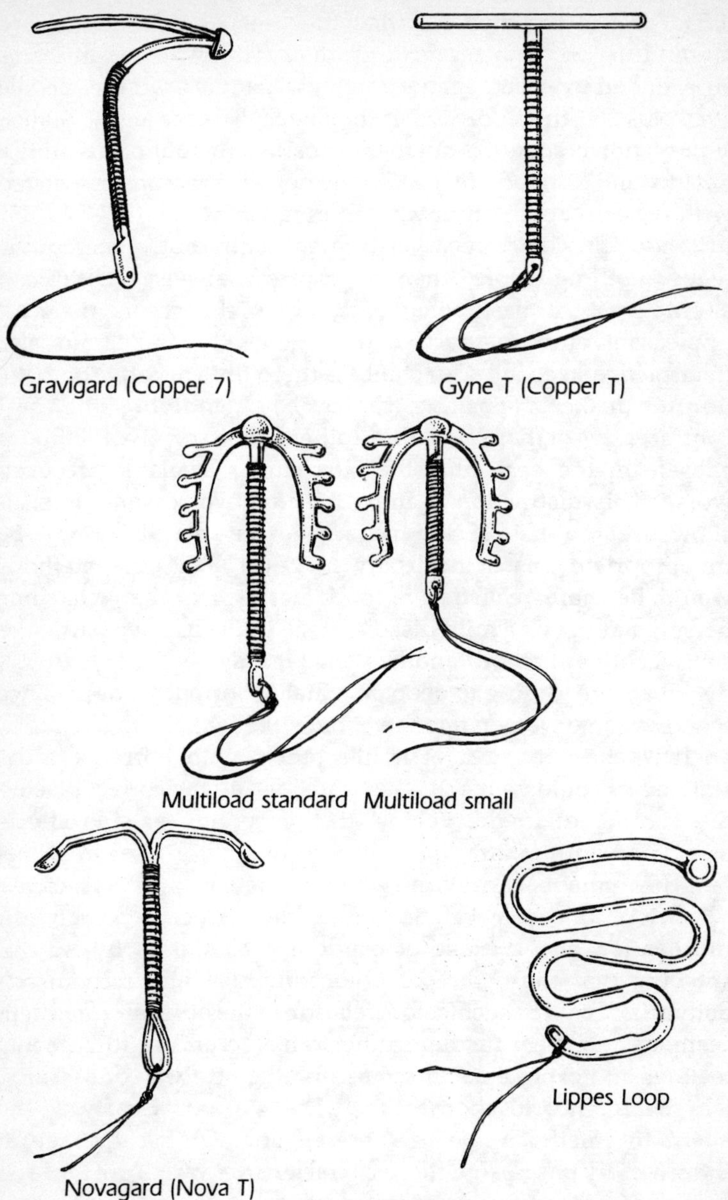

Figure 3 The six I.U.D.'s in common use today

The fact of the matter is that the use of any contraceptive method is an unpleasant business. The whole subject is surrounded by such negative feelings that it is a wonder people ever seek out the information they need. The reason why such information is sought is not for the positive reasons of ensuring a healthy and fulfilled life, but for the negative reasons associated with concern about an unwanted pregnancy.

It seems the choice between different contraceptive methods is really nothing more than a choice between unpleasant alternatives. At best, what each of us chooses is the *least* unpleasant and unattractive of a generally unpleasant and unattractive selection. Our choice is therefore a negative one. We do not make a positive choice by identifying the best contraceptive of those available; rather a contraceptive method is chosen on the basis that the alternatives available are even worse. This distinction is important for two reasons. First, it shows that a list of the advantages of the IUD may be inappropriate (a list of the disadvantages of all the other methods would be more realistic). Second, it suggests that what one person may see as a mild disadvantage in the use of a particular contraceptive method, another person may see as an extreme disadvantage leading to deep personal abhorrence. For instance whereas some women tolerate – but still dislike – the fitting of an IUD, the very idea of it fills others with horror. Similar statements could be made when considering the correct placing of spermicides in the vagina, the perception of side effects associated with taking the contraceptive pill, in the emotional fantasies about castration when considering a vasectomy operation, or even beliefs about the association between prostitution and the use of condoms. All this is by way of showing that the choice of a contraceptive method is often determined by a host of factors relating to the other, non-chosen, methods which in turn are interpreted according to personal feelings and experience. It seems that the best way of deciding whether or not to choose the IUD is to look closely at the alternative methods available and see if the IUD has the edge on the others by possessing those characteristics which are the least unpleasant for you at the present time.

So, when thinking about which contraceptive method to

choose, start by breaking down each of the available methods into its identifiable characteristics (what those of us doing research into this topic call its **'attributes'**). These characteristics or attributes describe a contraceptive method in terms of what behaviour is required for the use of the method to be effective. They include answers to such questions as:

i) Who uses it?
ii) When is it used?
   – before intercourse?
   – during intercourse?
   – after intercourse?
   – independent of intercourse?
iii) How is it used?
iv) What is involved in obtaining it?
v) What part of the body does it affect?
vi) What equipment goes with it?
vii) How is it stored when not in use?
viii) Where is it obtained?
ix) How much does it cost?
x) How effective is it in preventing pregnancy?
xi) What side effects are associated with it?
xii) How long do supplies last?

This list could be longer if more detail is required, but these twelve questions provide a good start. The next step is for the user to examine carefully her own situation, both at the present time and in the forseeable future. This can also be presented as a series of questions some of which may be of a highly personal kind, for example:

i) How old are you?
ii) Have you already had a baby?
iii) Is it your intention to have a baby in the future?
iv) Have you a history of medical problems associated with pregnancy?
v) Have you ever had medical problems of a gynaecological nature?
vi) Do you have one, or more, sexual partners?
vii) Are your sexual relationships of a stable kind?

viii) Would you find it difficult to discuss contraceptive methods with your partner?
ix) Do you smoke?

Again this list could be longer but the answers to these questions should provide sufficient information to reduce the number of alternative methods from which a final choice has to be made. If the IUD, the pill or the diaphragm are being considered, the final choice will doubtless follow a medical examination and a discussion about the likely method with a medical advisor. However, some of the more personal questions listed above are often not asked, even when medical advice is being sought. This lack of questioning may be due to a variety of reasons including the wish not to offend, but nevertheless most medical researchers agree that such questions are relevant. For example, the IUD should not normally be the first choice among women who are experiencing sexual relationships with more than one partner. While the IUD offers protection against an unwanted pregnancy it does not provide similar protection against pelvic infection and it is known that the incidence of pelvic infection rises as the number of sexual partners increases. In contrast, the condom or the diaphragm offers protection against both pregnancy and infection and in such circumstances may be a more appropriate method to choose (provided always that the other disadvantages of the condom or diaphragm use can be tolerated).

By looking both at the characteristics of the available methods of contraception, and bearing in mind your own personality and circumstances, you have a better chance of choosing a suitable and appropriate method. The following descriptions permit a rough comparison of the IUD with the other methods of contraception most commonly available in family planning clinics at the present time. Besides the methods discussed here, there are methods such as male and female sterilisation, withdrawal, spermicides, injectable hormones and the group of methods which come under the heading 'natural' family planning. Each has its advantages and disadvantages and can be assessed using a similar procedure.

CONDOM

The condom is a sheath of thin latex rubber material which covers the penis and prevents semen from entering the female reproductive tract.

Effectiveness	85-98% if a spermicide is used as well. Incorrect use (fitting too late, or removal too late allowing semen to escape) will increase the failure rate. Can be torn if carelessly handled.
Medical side effects	Virtually no unwanted side effects. Rare reports of allergy to rubber in men and women. Positive side effects reported include lower rates of sexually transmitted infections and of cervical cancer.
Used by	The man.
When used	During intercourse.
How used	Placed over the erect penis after foreplay.
Where obtained	Pharmacies, some barbers, slot machines, mail order, family planning clinics.
Frequency of supplies	Disposable. Easily obtainable.
Part of body affected	Penis. Some sensitivity may be lost.
Storage/ equipment	Easy to store. No equipment required.
Other issues	Interruption of lovemaking. Removal and disposal following sexual intercourse required.

DIAPHRAGM/CAP

The diaphragm is a flat, circular, flexible barrier, usually made of thin latex rubber and designed to carry a spermicidal cream, which covers the entrance to the uterus and prevents the entry of sperm.

Effectiveness	About 85-97%. Improper use (incorrect fitting or too early removal) will significantly reduce this figure.
Medical side effects	No unwanted side effects. Rare reports of allergy to rubber. Positive side effects include reports of a reduced incidence of cervical cancer.
Used by	The woman.
When used	Fitted before intercourse and left in place for several hours afterwards.
How used	Correct size of cap fitted by doctor or nurse. Woman taught how to apply spermicide and place cap in correct position. Requires practice and some skill in use.
Where obtained	Most family planning clinics and some general practitioners.
Frequency of supplies	Check on correct fit required from time to time; changes in body weight and other factors may affect size of diaphragm/cap needed. Not disposable; must be regularly checked for damage and replaced as necessary.
Part of body affected	Vagina.
Storage/ equipment	Stored in special container. Must be kept clean and dry when not in use.
Other issues	The messiness of fitting and removal appears to be the main disadvantage. No apparent interference with sexual sensitivity.

ORAL CONTRACEPTION (THE PILL)

Oral contraception is provided by tablets which contain varying amounts of oestrogen and/or progestogen hormones. These hormones affect the functioning of the reproductive system in a number of ways and prevent conception taking place.

Effectiveness	99%. This may be reduced with some low-dosage 'mini' pills if these are not taken absolutely regularly.
Medical side effects	Various. There are a number of medical contra-indications to pill use, and consultation with a doctor is necessary. Some adjustment of the type of pill taken may be required to avoid side effects such as nausea, weight gain, headaches. More serious side effects occasionally occur; these are associated with blood clotting. Pill use has also been linked with an increased risk of cancer of the cervix and breast.
Used by	The woman.
When used	Once daily. Some pills need to be taken every day and others allow a break of a few days once in every 28 days.
How used	Taken by mouth.
Where obtained	On medical prescription only. All family planning clinics and most general practitioners.
Frequency of supplies	Sufficient for three or six months use is usually prescribed.
Part of body affected	Generalised effect.
Storage/ equipment	Easy to store. No equipment required.
Other issues	Older women, and women who smoke, are more likely to suffer from the circulatory side effects of the pill.

INTRAUTERINE DEVICE (IUD/COIL/LOOP)

The IUD is a small object designed to be placed inside the uterus, and is made in a variety of shapes and sizes. It is usually made of plastic, sometimes with the addition of copper wire. How it prevents pregnancy is not fully understood, but is believed to affect the biochemistry of the uterus in some way.

Effectiveness	96-99%.
Medical side effects	Menstrual bleeding may become heavier and more painful. The device may be expelled from the uterus. There may be an increased likelihood of pelvic infection. There is a rare – but higher – risk of ectopic pregnancy in a woman who becomes pregnant whilst wearing an IUD. Rarely, the IUD may perforate through the uterine wall.
Used by	The woman.
When used	Permanently in place.
How used	Fitted by a doctor or nurse. No further action required.
Where obtained	Most family planning clinics and some general practitioners.
Frequency of supplies	Annual check-up is usually required. The device may remain in place for several years (10-15 years is not unusual) in the absence of side effects. Copper-bearing devices do require more frequent change.
Part of body affected	Uterus.
Storage/ equipment	None.
Other issues	Is effective against pregnancy immediately after fitting. Removal requires the assistance of a doctor or nurse.

CHAPTER 2

Personal factors to consider

Obviously the IUD will not suit every woman, nor is it necessarily the most suitable method of family planning to be used during all the years a woman might wish to be protected against an unwanted pregnancy. A method which might be suitable at one stage in a person's life may be inappropriate at another time which is why it is important to assess your own individual requirements when choosing a method of contraception. This applies as much to using an IUD as it does to any other method. For instance, changes occur in the size, shape and muscular tone of the uterus as a woman gets older and as she bears more children, which means that experience of IUD use will be different for women at different stages in their lives (see Figure 4). If a younger childless woman experiences an unacceptable side effect of IUD use – perhaps an unwanted pregnancy – then this experience may well put her off using an

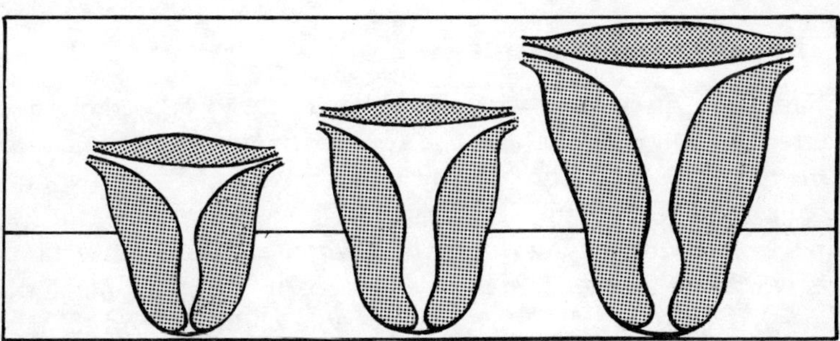

Figure 4 The difference in the size and shape of the uterus before and after having children
a) Young woman – no births **b)** Adult woman – no births **c)** Adult woman – previous births

IUD later on, at a stage in her life when the IUD would normally have been a good method to choose.

What might happen *after* IUD use is discontinued is also relevant and may be more important for some women than for others. For example, it is known that IUD use is associated with an increased (albeit small) risk of pelvic infection; such infection may be associated with greater difficulty in subsequently starting a pregnancy when this is desired. Whereas this news may not unduly concern older women who have had all the children they plan to have, the same could not be said for younger women who may be considering IUD use as a temporary measure before the planned birth of their first child. Adverse experiences resulting from the use of an IUD at an inappropriate time and in inappropriate circumstances will doubtless prejudice the person concerned for the rest of her life. Not only does this reduce the subsequent range of choices open to her, but the unfortunate experiences she (rightly) describes to others are likely to spread still further this reluctance about IUD use. Satisfied users seldom speak out about the advantages and benefits they see in their chosen contraceptive method; this leaves the field to the less than contented users. Perhaps this is as it should be for efforts should continually be made to remove all the disadvantages associated with the use of any contraceptive method, irrespective of the age and circumstances of the potential user.

The potential IUD user

There are three basic criteria which relate to acceptable and effective IUD use: the age, the parity (the number of full-term births), and the future reproductive intention of the woman concerned. The figures in Chapter 7 give the varying success rates of IUD use among women of different ages and parity, but it is worth noting here that differences are present. In general, the older IUD users who have two or more children tend to have fewer unacceptable side effects.

Reference to a potential IUD user's age and parity is not as simple as it may at first seem. When the assessment of IUDs first began during the 1960s, IUDs were generally only fitted among older married women who had already given birth to a child. It was not until the 1970s that younger women who had not had a baby began to be considered as suitable candidates for IUD use. As far as assessment of how effective the IUD is in preventing unwanted pregnancies, this had two important effects. First, women who had already given birth to a child were clearly fertile and able to have children when not using some form of contraception. Among a group of younger childless women who have not demonstrated their fertility, there will be a proportion who are unknowingly infertile and who will be unable to have a baby even if they were not using an IUD or some other form of contraception. This means that an IUD will look more effective than it really is if an assessment is made among women who have not yet proved that they are fertile. Studies among *parous* women then will provide a truer assessment of the IUD's ability to prevent an unwanted pregnancy.

But it is not so straightforward as this because *age* introduces a second, contradictory factor. Older women become progressively less likely to conceive even though they may have demonstrated their fertility by having a child at an earlier age. Taking these effects together – proven fertility and age – assessing the usefulness of an IUD becomes a complicated business. This does provide a warning that to be sure about the value or meaning of any information provided, one needs to look as closely at the type of woman wearing the IUD as at the IUD model itself. It is easy to show a very low pregnancy rate with a particular device if the women in the study are all childless and over the age of 35 years!

The term 'future reproductive intention' is a comparatively new one, introduced by the research team at Exeter University when it was found that just looking at a woman's age and parity was not enough to explain the varying reactions of women to the most common side effect associated with IUD use, that of an increase in the amount of menstrual bleeding. This side effect was often more important than all the other reasons put together in influencing women to request the removal of their IUDs. Both the age and parity of the IUD user appear to be related to reported incidents of this increased bleeding, but the *willingness* to discontinue use of the IUD as a consequence of increased bleeding appears to depend upon the woman's intentions with regard to whether or not she hopes to have another baby in the future, as well as by the options open to her in terms of switching to another contraceptive method. In the early 1970s it was reported in a large-scale American study that the incidence of unacceptable bleeding among IUD users decreased as the women became older. In the British study, women were asked directly about this problem and it was discovered that complaints about bleeding were no different among the older women than among the younger women. However, the younger women were more likely to consult the doctor who fitted the IUD and demand a removal of the device because of this side effect, whereas the older women were more likely to make no complaint and not to report the increase in bleeding. Many of the younger women explained that they were merely spacing pregnancies at the time and that while an unplanned pregnancy resulting from removal of the IUD would be inconvenient, it would not be disastrous for them. A change in method – or the use of no method at all – might result in the next pregnancy being earlier by a few months, but in any event it was their intention to have another baby. The older women tended to react in a very different way. These women had completed their families and were using IUDs as a means of ensuring that no more pregnancies would take place. Another pregnancy for such women would have serious repercussions on their lives, and the avoidance of pregnancy was extremely important to them. In addition, because of their age and the increased likelihood this brings of experiencing side effects from oral contraception, the option of changing to the pill was not available to them. The older IUD user it seems would prefer to put up with the nuisance of increased menstrual bleeding because an unwanted pregnancy would be an even greater problem. This difference in reaction to the occurrence of increased bleeding meant that when a statistical assessment took place, removal of the IUD following a complaint of increased bleeding was more likely to be seen among younger women, with an *apparent* reduction of the problem as the age of the women increased. This is not to say that all older IUD users make this choice, but sufficient of them do so to reduce the *reported* rate of increased bleeding among this particular group.

Put simply, older women were more likely to use the IUD to stop further pregnancies whereas younger women were more likely to use it to space pregnancies. Add to this the more recent category of IUD users who have not yet given birth to a child and three distinct categories of future pregnancy intention emerge: a woman may wish to *delay* the birth of her first child; a woman who has given birth to a child may wish to *space* the birth of future children; or a woman may have decided that her family is complete and that she now wishes to *stop* having children. (These three categories are often described in shorthand as 'delayers', 'spacers' and 'stoppers'.) Recognition of these three categories allows for greater understanding in the choice of an appropriate contraceptive method for each stage of family building. Clearly, undergoing male or female sterilisation is not a method available to those classed as 'delayers' or 'spacers'; nor should a method which possesses a relatively high risk of pregnancy be chosen by women who would define themselves as 'stoppers'.

The age, parity and future reproductive intention of the potential IUD user are all related to each other. Although the 'delayer' is childless, some childless women are also 'stoppers' in that they have decided that they will never want a baby in the future. Parous women may be either 'spacers' or 'stoppers' depending on their desire for a future pregnancy. This emphasis on reproductive intention is important because no method of contraception is 100 per cent effective in preventing pregnancy, and the acceptability of different levels of risk of pregnancy is clearly related to whether or not a pregnancy may be desired at some time in the future. The categories of 'delayer', 'spacer' and 'stopper' introduce an element of motivation into the use of the IUD, and the toleration of side effects associated with its use. Medical, social and personal risks associated with an unplanned and unwanted pregnancy often outweigh the disadvantages of wearing an IUD, even among those women for whom the IUD may not be considered the wisest choice. It is apparent that there can be no hard and fast rules about who should and who should not wear an IUD. Higher risks may be associated with other alternative methods, and personal circumstances, especially as these relate to the degree of support received from a sexual partner, may be of overriding importance. With this in mind the following summaries, distilled from eighteen years research experience, are offered.

The woman who has not had a previous pregnancy

With the development of IUDs which could be loaded into a narrow inserter, it was claimed that a woman who had not yet had a baby could now be fitted with an IUD just as easily as a woman who had already given birth to children. Where a pregnancy and birth has not occurred, the muscle of the uterus is unstretched and the openings at either end of the cervical canal tend to be tighter. To pass an IUD through the cervical canal was often more difficult in such cases and discomfort was often experienced at the time of fitting. The development of small-bore inserters has certainly permitted the more common fitting of IUDs among childless women, but it would be incorrect to claim that discomfort at the time of fitting has been entirely removed. Discomfort at fitting is undoubtedly greater for the childless woman than for one who has borne children in recent years. There are obvious physical reasons for this, but psychological factors are also present. Most women, prior to the birth of their first child, have not usually experienced the type of genital manipulation the fitting of an IUD requires. It is understandable that there is considerable tenseness and apprehension. A tightening of the already taut muscles of the pelvic floor takes place in such circumstances and makes the fitting of an IUD even more uncomfortable than it otherwise might be. Competent clinic staff and doctors do their best to create a relaxed atmosphere and in this they are often successful. Nevertheless, an IUD fitting, at the best of times, could not be called a pleasant experience and those undergoing it for the first time are particularly vulnerable. The good doctor will tell a woman in advance exactly what is entailed in fitting an IUD, as well as discussing with her the advantages and disadvantages of IUD use in general terms. For a number of years the Exeter research team has been advising that the IUD should not be the first choice of contraceptive method for childless women, and serious consideration should be given by these women to alternative methods of contraception. In addition to the device being more difficult to fit the following points should also be considered by the childless woman:

1) The pregnancy risk is higher than with most oral contraceptives and is also higher than among women who are using IUDs and who have borne children.
2) The likelihood of expulsion of the IUD from the uterus tends to be higher than among women who have borne children. This finding may be related to the increased pregnancy rate; for expulsion to take place, displacement of the device within the uterus must first have occurred, so reducing the protection against pregnancy.
3) There is a small increased risk of pelvic inflammatory disease among IUD users and this can lead to subsequent infertility. This increased risk is greater in younger childless women wearing an IUD.

In addition it should be emphasised that the IUD offers no protection against infection (as do some other contraceptive methods). Recent studies have shown that there is a link between the number of sexual partners and the level of risk of pelvic infection which may lead on to infertility: the greater the number of sexual partners the greater is the risk of pelvic infection and subsequent infertility. Despite the listing of these disadvantages, it would be incorrect to suggest that nulliparous women should never consider the use of an IUD; much will depend on the medical, social and personal circumstances of the person concerned, and the contraceptive alternatives available at the time.

The woman with one or more children

Women who have had children are good candidates for IUD use. There is a small chance of pregnancy occurring after an IUD has been fitted, but this risk tends to lessen with increasing age and as fecundity is reduced. Most research on IUDs has been undertaken using information collected from among parous women of varying ages. For convenience, IUD users who have borne children are considered to be of **low parity** if they have had one or two children and of **high parity** if they have had three or more children. Again, the potential IUD user should be seen in the context of her future reproductive intention; the parous woman who is spacing pregnancies will have differing needs from the parous woman who is certain she wants no future pregnancy.

The woman of low parity (1 or 2 births) who is spacing pregnancies

These are the ideal candidates for IUD use. A small risk of an unplanned pregnancy is present, but this is less of a problem than it would be for those who definitely did not want another pregnancy. Care must be taken that future fertility is not affected in any way. This means seeking prompt medical attention if any signs of possible pelvic infection appear.

The woman of low parity (1 or 2 births) who wants no further pregnancy

The risk of pregnancy suggests that a woman in this group is not quite so suitable as the parous woman who is spacing pregnancies. It should be noted that this risk of pregnancy is very small (see Chapter 5) and that age plays an important part in defining this level of risk. By and large, the older woman has lower fecundity than the younger woman and the risk of pregnancy is likely to be low. However, it is easy to describe this as a low risk when assessing the experience of unplanned pregnancies across hundreds or thousands of such IUD users, but the personal upset is still very distressing for the individual IUD user concerned. If a future pregnancy is definitely not desired, perhaps a more permanent method of contraception (such as male or female sterilisation) should be given consideration.

The woman of high parity (3 births and over) who is spacing pregnancies

Again, these are ideal candidates for IUD use. A small risk of pregnancy persists. All available evidence suggests that the chance of expulsion of the device from the uterus, and the reported incidence of discomfort associated with heavier menstrual bleeding, are both reduced compared with the experience of IUD users of lower parity.

The woman of high parity (3 births and over) who wants no further pregnancy

The same points arise here as for the woman of lower parity who definitely does not want another pregnancy. The risk of pregnancy remains, but the fact of high parity suggests that the women concerned are very fertile and that if anyone is likely to become pregnant, women in this group are likely to do so. To redress this imbalance, women of high parity are also usually older women which means that their fecundity is likely to be reduced. But younger women under the age of 30 years who have experienced three or more full-term pregnancies are particularly vulnerable and more permanent methods of contraception should be given consideration. If male or female sterilisation is not acceptable and the IUD is chosen, then a spermicidal cream or pessary could be used as an additional safeguard.

The woman who has recently experienced the birth of a child

An IUD may be fitted within a few hours of the birth of a child. There are obvious advantages of having an IUD fitted at this time, but additional care needs to be taken. The major problems of IUDs fitted at this time are the high level of expulsion of the device from the uterus and an increased risk of the device perforating the uterine wall. This is due to the rapidly changing shape, structure and muscle tone of the uterus during the post-natal period. Doctors are aware of these additional problems and this partly explains why immediate post-partum fitting of IUDs is not more common. Some researchers believe that waiting for up to 12 hours after the birth will reduce the likelihood of IUD expulsion. Most doctors agree that fittings should not take place between the end of the first week and up to six weeks after delivery. If fitted early after the birth, it seems that the careful placing of the device within the uterus is more important than the type of device used. A variety of devices have been developed specifically for post-partum fitting, but these are not generally available, being confined in the main for use in family planning programmes in developing countries.

A second optimal time for IUD fitting occurs about six weeks after delivery. This will coincide with the scheduled post-natal examination. The chances of expulsion and perforation of the uterus are by this stage much reduced, and mothers being fitted with an IUD at this time are at no greater risk of unwanted side effects than other IUD users who have not recently experienced a pregnancy. This is a more popular time for IUD fitting because it avoids interfering with the more important experiences which inevitably surround the mother at the time her baby is born. The need to provide an IUD immediately after delivery has advantages in those situations when this is the only time the mother is likely to attend a hospital or clinic, but this hardly applies in developed countries. The advice of most medical and research teams is to wait for about six to twelve weeks after the birth of a baby before making an appointment for an IUD fitting. If the woman is breastfeeding during this time, this does provide some contraceptive protection, although the exact mechanism by which breastfeeding exerts its antifertility effect is not fully known. It is thought to depend to some extent on the frequency and regularity of the feeds, and particularly as to whether these continue during the night also. But breastfeeding cannot be relied upon completely to prevent another pregnancy. This means that some form of temporary contraceptive protection is needed during this interim period.

The woman who has recently experienced an abortion

Several studies have shown that among women who have recently experienced an early miscarriage, or who have had an abortion during the first twelve weeks of pregnancy, the fitting of an IUD creates no special problems. There is no likelihood of an increased risk of complications at the time of fitting or immediately afterwards, although there are some reports of the early return of menstruation with slightly heavier bleeding than usual. Researchers emphasise that there is no increased risk of uterine infection among such women; no significant difference has been found in subsequent unintended pregnancy or other unwanted side effects, when compared with women who experience the more routine fitting of an IUD.

The fitting of an IUD in women who have experienced a miscarriage or abortion later on in pregnancy – that is after the first twelve weeks – requires the same care and consideration as the post-natal fitting of an IUD. The difference between IUD fitting and use after early abortion and after a full-term birth is related almost exclusively to the differences in the size, shape and muscular condition of the uterus. If a late miscarriage or abortion has occurred, available evidence suggests it would be wise to wait for about six to twelve weeks before the IUD is fitted. This gives time for the uterus to return to normal and also provides time for the resolution of any other immediate or psychological effects of the abortion experience.

The woman who has just experienced sexual intercourse without contraceptive protection

Some years ago, when pressed to describe the best available contraceptive, a pioneering doctor who began her family planning work in the West Country as early as 1930, replied 'Two sensible people.' When amplifying this short answer, she pointed out that these two people engaging in a sexual relationship with each other would have agreed that on this occasion their sexual activity was, or was not, intended to lead to an attempted pregnancy. If pregnancy was not desired then some decisions had to be made about adequate and mutually acceptable contraceptive protection. This widely experienced family planning doctor recognised that this was an ideal situation which often does not happen in practice. Unprotected sexual intercourse, even when a pregnancy is the last thing a couple wants, frequently takes place. This absence of protection can be due to lack of planning and thought for future consequences, or simple forgetfulness. The non-availability of a suitable contraceptive, mistakes in contraceptive use or calculation, or the poor quality of the contraceptive itself are other reasons why unprotected sexual intercourse sometimes takes place.

The emergency post-coital fitting of an IUD has now become a recognised treatment in the prevention of an unintended pregnancy following an isolated act of unprotected intercourse. In such cases, where it is known there is a risk of pregnancy, the fitting of an IUD offers a high level of protection. In order to conform with the abortion law of the United Kingdom, the Department of Health advises that IUDs used in this way should be fitted within *five* days of the unprotected intercourse. The use of an IUD in such circumstances is based on the knowledge that the ovum, if fertilised, takes a minimum time interval of about three days to reach the uterus from the fallopian tubes. The presence of an IUD in the uterus will stop the fertilised ovum from implanting into the uterine wall and pregnancy is therefore prevented from taking place. If implantation had taken place any subsequent fitting of an IUD could be classed as an action likely to procure an abortion. It is for this reason that the three day restriction on the post-coital fitting of an IUD is officially recognised. It is worth remembering that many acts of sexual intercourse where contraception is not used do not result in a pregnancy. One author has estimated that on a day randomly selected during the menstrual cycle, the odds of a pregnancy resulting from unprotected sexual intercourse is about 1 in 33. However, it should be noted that these odds increase dramatically to about 1 in 4 if sexual intercourse takes place shortly before ovulation. At what time in the menstrual cycle the unprotected intercourse takes place therefore becomes an important factor in deciding whether or not to seek medical advice. Some doctors have suggested that if unprotected sexual intercourse has taken place and a pregnancy is to be avoided, action is only required if the sexual activity occurred around the middle of the menstrual cycle, that is at the time when ovulation is likely to have occurred and therefore the woman is at her most fertile stage.

The use of the IUD as a post-coital method of contraception has the added advantage that it will continue to be effective as a more planned means of contraception until it is removed. Not only is the IUD helping to treat an immediate problem, but it also continues to offer protection over an extended period of time. If an IUD is fitted as a post-coital measure, the incidence and likelihood of side effects are exactly the same as for other users of similar age and parity.

CHAPTER 3

Medical factors to consider

There are a number of medical factors which a doctor must consider before deciding whether or not to advise use of an IUD. These medical factors may be important either individually or in combination with each other. Most doctors will know of a number of medical conditions which would suggest the IUD should not normally be used. These medical conditions are known as **contra-indications** (i.e. indications against) and are usually divided into two categories. The first category is of **absolute contra-indications**: these are conditions or diseases which indicate that a woman who is suffering from such a condition or disease should *definitely* not be fitted with an IUD. One example of this would be if the woman had a suspected malignancy of the reproductive tract. The risks of IUD use in such cases would outweigh any possible advantage wearing an IUD might bring. Alternatively the presence of certain conditions could lead the doctor to contravene the law or accepted medical practice if an IUD were fitted; for example, if the woman was known or believed to be pregnant at the time. Both these examples are absolute contra-indications to IUD use.

However, there are other medical conditions which, whilst sometimes being a reason for not fitting an IUD, are not an absolute bar to such fitting. The medical conditions in this second category are called **relative contra-indications**. In these cases the risk of IUD use has to be weighed against the disadvantages of *not* fitting an IUD. Most doctors would agree that where an anatomical, structural abnormality of the uterus is discovered an IUD may not be the most appropriate method of contraception to use; but this will depend on the type and severity of the abnormality. Uterine abnormality is therefore a relative contra-indication and not an absolute contra-indication to IUD fitting. This division into categories of absolute and relative contra-indication is to some extent an artificial division. Whilst almost all doctors may be agreed that a small number of specific conditions constitute a complete bar to IUD fitting, there may be less agreement about the conditions which provide a *relative* contra-indication to IUD use: what one doctor considers to be a relative contra-indication may be considered an absolute contra-indication by another doctor. Equally what may be considered a relative contra-indication in the case of one particular woman may be considered an absolute contra-indication in the circumstances of another woman.

The evaluation and balancing of the potential benefits and potential hazards of IUD use is complex, and an individual decision must be made in each case. Not only must the risks and benefits of IUD use be balanced, but the potential hazards of other alternative methods of contraception must also be taken into consideration, as well as the demands and problems of an unintended pregnancy. From this it can be seen that the doctors who fit IUDs have to make judgements which are sometimes not easy to make. Both the personal life of the woman who is considering the fitting of an IUD, and also the relative weight that should be placed on any reported medical condition must be carefully considered. The doctor has to be concerned with the whole woman who is to be fitted with the IUD rather than only with the technical problem of inserting an IUD into a uterus.

The medical conditions discussed below are those which should be considered by the doctor contemplating the fitting of an IUD. (These refer to pre-existing medical conditions only. Whether or not an IUD is fitted will still depend upon the results of a physical examination even if the medical history appears satisfactory.)

Absolute medical contra-indications to IUD use

Current or repeated history of pelvic infection

This infection can spread from the uterus to affect the fallopian tubes and the ovaries and is usually described by the single term 'pelvic inflammatory disease'. The infection is not necessarily sexually transmitted but in some instances it can be. The infection can vary in severity, and when mild may be difficult to diagnose with any certainty. In a severe attack the woman will have a fever and feel ill; she may have heavy or abnormal vaginal bleeding and complain of pain low in the abdomen; there will be tenderness of the reproductive organs and a vaginal examination may be painful. A woman who is currently being treated for any infection of the reproductive tract should not be fitted with an IUD. The IUD would be a foreign body in the uterus, and the presence of a foreign body aggravates an infection and prevents the body's natural defences from being effective. Similarly, where there is a medical history of repeated episodes of pelvic infection, even though infection is currently not present, an IUD should not be fitted. If a further attack occurred after IUD fitting, the presence of an IUD would be likely to exacerbate the problem and increase the severity of the attack.

The concern about the link between pelvic infection and IUD use is one that is raised frequently. Pelvic infection can damage the delicate structures of the reproductive system in a variety of ways and this damage frequently causes a reduction in fertility, with the result that a woman may not be able to become pregnant when she wishes to start a family at a future time. This topic is discussed in more detail in Chapter 5 where the relationship between IUD use and pelvic infection is examined fully. (Any experience of abnormal discharge, abnormal bleeding or pain and tenderness in the pelvic region should be brought to the attention of a doctor, irrespective of whether or not an IUD fitting is being contemplated.)

Known or suspected pregnancy

If there is any suspicion that a pregnancy has been established, an IUD should not be fitted. The fitting of an IUD under such circumstances could be construed as an attempt to terminate the pregnancy illegally and a doctor who knowingly did this would be contravening the law. This is one of the reasons why fitting the IUD either during or shortly after the end of a menstrual period is usually recommended. At such times there is no likelihood that a conception has already occurred.

This should not be confused with the legitimate post-coital fitting of an IUD within five days of an isolated, unprotected act of sexual intercourse (see Chapter 2). Reasonable suspicion that a pregnancy may have occurred requires more time than three days; a missed menstrual period following an occasion when unprotected sexual intercourse is known to have taken place is usually regarded as the minimum evidence for a reasonable suspicion of pregnancy.

Known or suspected cancer affecting the reproductive tract

There is no evidence whatsoever that IUD use can cause cancer of the reproductive system. However, where a malignancy is already present, or is suspected, an IUD should not be fitted; it is possible that the presence of an IUD could aggravate the condition. A previous history of a successfully treated cancer does not necessarily exclude an IUD fitting, but the family planning doctor may well arrange for a consultation with a gynaecologist for further assessment before attempting IUD fitting. Women who have had treatment following a positive cervical smear result are not debarred from having an IUD fitted, though again if the doctor is in any doubt a consultation with the gynaecologist who carried out treatment may be arranged.

Relative contra-indications to IUD use, and other conditions where additional care is required

Anaemia

An IUD should not be fitted until the type and cause of the anaemia has been determined, and the condition has been successfully treated. Heavy periods are a common cause of anaemia in women. The reason for avoiding IUD fitting is because use of the IUD is known to increase the amount of menstrual blood loss. If there is already a problem of anaemia, then to use a contraceptive method which increases blood loss is obviously unwise. An alternative method of contraception should be used temporarily until the anaemia has been treated.

Rheumatic heart disease; congenital heart disease; renal disease

As has already been described, IUD use is associated with an increased risk of pelvic infection. If this infection were to enter the blood stream, it could have serious consequences for women who have a history of these diseases. Alternative methods of contraception should be considered by these women.

Heavy menstrual bleeding; irregular menstrual bleeding

Where irregular or heavy menstrual bleeding is taking place an IUD should not be fitted until the cause of these conditions has been determined, and the condition treated. Not only could the IUD exacerbate an existing problem, but the abnormal bleeding may be indicating the need for treatment of a more serious medical condition. This is not to say that the occasional occurrence of heavy, irregular or abnormal bleeding is always associated with a serious disorder, but it is wise to have this diagnosed and treated before an IUD fitting takes place. If no other method is acceptable, an IUD could be fitted but close medical supervision will be needed.

Abnormal vaginal discharge

Almost all women experience a vaginal discharge of some sort, but if this is considered to be abnormal, then it should be brought to the attention of a doctor. In such cases it would be unwise for an IUD to be fitted until the discharge had been treated and cleared up. The discharge might be due to an infection, and the organisms could be spread up into the uterus by the insertion of an IUD. This would spread the infection and possibly cause an attack of pelvic inflammatory disease.

Previous experience of pelvic infection

If pelvic infection is currently being treated or if there is a history of many episodes of such infection, an IUD should not be fitted. But there are situations in which doctors may fit an IUD even though an attack of pelvic infection has taken place sometime in the past. Fittings could take place if there has been only a limited experience of infection, where its occurrence was confined to one or two isolated incidents. Some medical teams require that any previous incident must have been completely cleared up for not less than three months before the IUD fitting. Where an isolated incident has taken place within the last three months, delay in IUD fitting is normally recommended. This applies equally if previous infection has been associated with a full-term birth or a miscarriage. If an IUD is fitted where there is a history of pelvic infection, the woman should be conscientious about attending for check-ups and should report any subsequent signs of infection without delay.

Severe dysmenorrhoea (painful periods)

As well as increasing the amount of blood loss during a period, periods also sometimes become more painful after IUD fitting. If a woman already experiences very painful periods, these might be made even worse by IUD use.

Fibroids

Fibroids are benign (i.e. non-cancerous) growths of the uterine wall. These growths cause enlargement or distortion of the uterus and often also cause heavy menstrual bleeding. The IUD is inappropriate for women with large or multiple fibroids because these would make insertion more difficult and increase the risk of the device perforating the uterine wall. The incidence of side effects, such as expulsion and increased menstrual bleeding, is also likely to be greater.

Structural abnormalities of the uterus

There is considerable variation in the size, shape and position of the 'normal' uterus, but sometimes these variations are sufficiently great to be classed as 'abnormal'. This is one of the reasons why a pelvic examination is necessary at the time of IUD fitting. Rarely, the uterus may be partially divided into two sections. In order to be effective in preventing pregnancy an IUD has to be carefully placed at the top (or 'fundus') of the uterus. If this proper placement is prevented by structural abnormalities of the uterus, then the protection afforded against pregnancy may be greatly reduced. The likelihood of the IUD perforating the uterine wall is also increased.

Previous operations on the uterus, (including caesarian section)

It is possible that where there is scarring and consequent weakness of the uterine wall following an operation, the likelihood of an IUD perforating the wall of the uterus is greater. However, this seems to be more of a theoretical than a practical possibility, and most doctors do not consider a previous caesarian section operation to be a contra-indication to IUD use. Previous operations on the cervix may cause scarring which may make the cervical canal narrower and more rigid. Because the IUD has to pass through the cervical canal, this narrowing and lack of flexibility may make insertion more difficult and consequently more painful. Where there is any doubt about the advisability of fitting an IUD, a doctor may advise referral to a gynaecologist.

Copper allergy

Most of the recently developed IUDs contain the addition of copper wire which is wound around the plastic stem of the device. Women who possess a known allergy to copper (or who suffer from Wilson's disease – a very rare, inherited disorder of copper excretion) should therefore not be fitted with these newer copper-bearing IUDs. Inert, plastic devices without the addition of copper are still available and women who are allergic to copper may safely use these inert devices. (See Chapter 7 for a detailed description of different IUD models.)

Previous ectopic pregnancy

An ectopic pregnancy is one which develops *outside* the uterus, usually in the fallopian tube. The risk of an ectopic pregnancy among IUD users who inadvertently become pregnant whilst wearing an IUD is known to be higher than among pregnant women generally. All IUD users who suspect they may have become pregnant should seek medical advice at once, but this is particularly important in the case of women who have a history of ectopic pregnancy (see also Chapter 5).

Ongoing drug treatment

When deciding whether or not an IUD is an appropriate method of contraception, the family planning doctor needs to know about any medication which is currently being taken by the woman.

The amount of menstrual blood loss is known to increase following the fitting of an IUD. In a woman currently taking **anti-coagulant** drugs, the amount of increased blood loss may become unacceptable.

Steroid drugs have the effect of reducing inflammatory reaction in body tissues. This means that if a woman currently taking steroids develops a pelvic infection, this condition may be masked and may become severe and well established before producing any symptoms.

Diabetes

There have been reports suggesting that there is a higher risk of accidental pregnancy while wearing an IUD among insulin-dependent diabetic women. Other studies have found no such difference, and have reported that diabetic IUD users appear to run no additional risk. In 1982 the medical advisory panel of the Family Planning Association looked carefully at all the available information, and came to the conclusion that present evidence does not justify a recommendation that diabetic women should not be fitted with an IUD. There is, nevertheless, a need for caution, and the woman should be conscientious about attending for check-ups and should report any untoward symptoms at once.

Epilepsy

It has been reported that an epileptic seizure can occur at the time of IUD fitting in women who suffer from epilepsy. There is no evidence that IUD fitting acts as a trigger in causing an epileptic attack, and the connection between the two events may be coincidental. However, the doctor fitting the IUD should be informed if a woman suffers from epilepsy, in order to ensure the best possible care in the unlikely event of an attack occurring.

CHAPTER 4

Having an IUD fitted

Once you have decided to use an IUD as a method of contraception, the next step is to decide where to get the device fitted and to arrange an appointment at an appropriate time. The question of where to seek IUD fitting depends upon the more fundamental issue of who is the most appropriate person to fit the IUD.

Who is the best person to fit an IUD?

This is not such an easy question to answer as might appear at first. Much will depend on the skills of the person fitting the IUD, the type of IUD being fitted, the circumstances of the woman being fitted, and, perhaps above all, the confidence that the woman has in the person carrying out the fitting. The IUD Research Network has been collecting information about IUD fitting and use throughout the UK since the beginning of the 1970s. This research has shown very clearly that the person who fits the IUD is just as important as the type of IUD which is fitted. Most research studies compare the performance of one type of IUD model with that of other types of IUD models, and report which model has the lowest pregnancy rate, or the lowest incidence of expulsion or increased bleeding. However Research Network studies have shown that there can be a greater variation in the incidence of side effects between different clinics than between different IUD models: that is, a device which shows a pregnancy rate of say 1 per cent when fitted by a doctor in one clinic might show a pregnancy rate of 4 per cent when fitted by another doctor in another clinic. This may well be because of differences in the groups of women which the two clinics serve; but undoubtedly the skill and the experience of the different doctors also figures very largely in influencing the results.

One problem is that in the UK at the present time there is no formal requirement that doctors should be specifically trained to fit IUDs. Many senior members of the medical profession, and especially those who take a particular interest in family planning services, are keen to see such training become mandatory. They believe IUD fittings should only be undertaken by doctors who have received a certificate of competence and are thereby registered to fit IUDs. As the fitting of an IUD is a minor operative procedure this seems a reasonable requirement. The Family Planning Association has estimated that of the 26,000 general practitioners in this country about 9,000 have undergone formal training in the fitting and follow-up of IUDs. These figures may be misleading in that among a group of doctors working together in a single large practice, the fitting of IUDs and the care of IUD users may have been entrusted to one or two members of the group who have undergone training, leaving the others to specialise in different areas of work.

However, training is not the only factor which affects the efficiency of IUD fitting. Medicine is a wide-ranging and demanding profession and many different types of skills are needed by doctors who choose to work in its various specialisations. Just as not all doctors would consider that they had the degree of manual dexterity needed to become a surgeon, so not all doctors have in equal amount the skills of manual dexterity which are needed for IUD fitting. Not only this but, once acquired, skills must be practised regularly if the degree of skill is to be maintained. It would appear then that the doctors most likely to have good results in IUD fitting will have been fully trained by an already experienced doctor; will have achieved a considerable degree of skill in carrying out this procedure; and will in the course of his or her routine work fit IUDs regularly and frequently to maintain this high level of skill.

It was noted earlier (in Chapter 2) that when assessing the performance of any particular IUD model, it was as important to look as closely at the type of woman wearing the IUD as at the IUD model itself. It is also true that the characteristics of the person who fits the IUD will have an effect on the outcome of that fitting. It would take a brave woman to confront her doctor with the question, 'How many IUDs have you fitted during the last month?' and to decline the fitting if the answer indicated very few! However, the choice of the doctor who is going to fit her IUD is an important choice, and a woman would be well advised to choose someone who specialises in this field. Perhaps the most sensible approach would be to ask for a preliminary discussion about all the possible types of family planning methods at the first appointment with the doctor, so that detailed questions about possible IUD use could be asked in the absence of any embarrassment.

Occasionally IUDs are fitted by specially trained nurses. Studies have been carried out in a number of countries where IUD fittings by doctors have been compared with fittings undertaken by nurses. Reports of these studies indicate that the nurses have as good a record as that of the doctors. In some instances nurses have been even more successful than doctors in terms of the subsequent experience of the IUD user. This could well be because the doctor is dealing with the more difficult cases and the nurse is only undertaking the more routine, straightforward fittings. The skill and judgement needed to deliver a baby is just as complex, perhaps more so, than that needed for IUD fitting; it therefore seems logical that midwives or other specially trained nurses should be used in this way.

When should an IUD be fitted?

An IUD can be fitted at any time during the menstrual cycle, but doctors usually advise fitting either during menstruation or very soon after bleeding has ceased. There are three reasons for this:

i) the IUD is easier to fit at this time and this in turn reduces the possibility of discomfort for the woman. This is because the cervix is softer and more malleable at this stage in the menstrual cycle;

ii) any small amount of blood loss due to the fitting of the IUD will not be noticeable;

iii) the menstrual period will confirm that conception has not occurred. An IUD must not be fitted if a pregnancy is suspected.

However, this ideal time for IUD fitting is not always achieved in practice. The appointment systems used in family planning clinics and the difficulty many women have in arranging a time when they are not either working or caring for small children means that such precise timing is often impossible. In addition, some women would definitely prefer not to attend at this time as they would be embarrassed by the prospect of an internal examination during a period. For these administrative and personal reasons IUD fittings tend to take place at any time that can conveniently be arranged. However, fitting at mid-cycle around the time of ovulation is often more difficult and can be more painful, and therefore is best avoided. This applies to all women, but particularly to women who have not borne children or who have just come off the pill. The cervix and cervical canal is more rigid at this time and is more likely to go into spasm during the fitting procedure.

A recent large-scale study demonstrated that it made no difference whether an IUD was fitted during (or soon after) menstruation in terms of the risk of pregnancy or expulsion or other side effects of IUD use. In its guidelines to doctors, the Department of Health recommends that IUD fitting should be undertaken as early in the menstrual cycle as possible and before day 20 unless alternative contraception has been used during the current menstrual cycle. These suggestions are given with the aim of avoiding fitting an IUD if there is a possibility that the woman has already conceived. Much will depend upon the clinical judgement of the doctor who is to fit the IUD, and few doctors would feel justified in asking a woman to return on a second occasion for IUD fitting without good reason.

Making an appointment

Most women who are considering having an IUD fitted will know of a medical practice where advice about the various contraceptive methods can be obtained. It may be that IUDs are also fitted at this practice but if this is not the case, a consultation at a family planning clinic will need to be arranged. It is also possible to approach a family planning clinic directly without first consulting your own general practitioner; the address and telephone number of your nearest clinic can be found in the telephone directory.

When making an appointment the receptionist will probably ask you if a general consultation is required, or if you have already decided on a particular method. If the appointment is for IUD fitting, the receptionist will almost certainly ask for the date on which your last menstrual period commenced, so it is useful to have this ready. This is also a good time to ask any general questions you may have: for example, are you likely to have to wait; how long will the whole procedure take; is there any provision for the care of small children; will you see a male or female doctor?

Be prepared

An internal examination will be necessary before an IUD is fitted. The bladder must be empty in order for the doctor to carry out this examination satisfactorily, so visit the lavatory just beforehand.

It is probably wiser to wear a skirt rather than trousers when attending for IUD fitting. Tights and pants will have to be removed and if trousers are worn these will have to be removed too leaving you feeling a little naked from the waist down. A skirt or dress provides more covering when getting up on to the high examination couch, and can be hitched up and still give partial covering during the examination and IUD fitting.

At the clinic

The first member of the team you are most likely to meet when attending a family planning clinic for IUD fitting is a clerk who will record basic information needed to maintain the necessary records. She will ask for your name, address, date of birth and also the name and address of your family doctor. (The clinic will normally write routinely to your family doctor informing him of the clinic consultation and IUD fitting.) It is this basic record which provides evidence for compilation of service statistics and for the administration of follow-up appointments in the future. Most clinic records are only kept for about two years after the woman concerned ceases to attend the clinic. Family doctors and private physicians often keep records for longer periods.

After completing the initial formalities, you may have to wait before the next phase of the consultation takes place. Sometimes this wait can be lengthy, depending on the amount of additional time required by those with earlier appointments. It is wise to take something to do; the magazines left out in the waiting room may be old and out of date. It is also wise to inform any companion who may have provided transport, or come to provide moral support, that the length of time an appointment will take is often unpredictable, mainly because of this waiting period.

The next person you will see will be the nurse who will record the more medically related information which is needed by the doctor fitting the IUD. This questioning will mainly be about previous pregnancies, including the dates and details of any known complications. A menstrual history will also be taken with particular emphasis on the amount, regularity and duration of your recent periods. If you have already chosen to use an IUD, the nurse may give you a leaflet which describes the IUD to be fitted. You will be given an opportunity to read this and then any questions which arise can be brought up with the doctor.

When you see the doctor he or she will ask about your previous medical history, about any health problems you may have at the present time, and about any medication you may be taking. There will also be an opportunity to ask questions and discuss any uncertainties you may have. This opportunity should not be ignored. It has already been emphasised that the successful use of an IUD not only requires a good product, but also a supportive relationship between the IUD user and the person responsible for the IUD fitting. A trusting relationship should be created at this first meeting and a frank discussion about the advantages and disadvantages of IUD use is an important part of this process.

Counselling by the doctor

Most IUD training manuals emphasise the need for the doctor to counsel the potential IUD user very carefully if successful use of the IUD is to take place. Ideally the doctor should:

i) describe the general advantages and disadvantages of IUD use, and the characteristics of the IUD model to be fitted;
ii) provide information about the procedures to be followed in the IUD fitting;
iii) explain the need for follow-up visits and the type of supervision which will be required.

It is important for the IUD user to know the name of the IUD model she is wearing. IUDs come in different shapes and sizes and have differing effects; knowing the name of the IUD being worn may save considerable anxiety at a later date. Popular reference to the 'coil' relates to the Saf-T-Coil, a device which was frequently used in Europe and America during the 1960s and 1970s. Its use has declined in recent years and it is now no longer manufactured. The name still clings though and many doctors, journalists and women wearing an IUD still erroneously refer to all IUDs as the 'coil'. The 'loop' is still with us, although its share of the IUD market is now only a fraction of what it was in the 1960s. The full name is the Lippes Loop, after its inventor Dr Jack Lippes, an American family planning doctor. Of all devices, the Lippes Loop has been the most widely used in the world, but the chances of a European or American woman actually wearing the 'loop' now are comparatively small.

It is surprising how many IUD users are unaware of the type and size of the IUD model they are wearing. To call all IUDs by the general name of a device which is now no longer available can create uncertainty and anxiety. If there is adverse publicity about a particular device, and women do not know the name of the device which they are wearing, they can be caused unnecessary worry. There have been two examples of IUD recall in recent years. The Hong Kong Triangle (or Ahmed's device) was found to contain an inferior quality of plastic which in some cases fragmented in the uterus. Only a few hundred devices had been fitted and all were eventually safely removed, but the anxiety generated among women wearing other IUDs (but who were not sure which device) created a great deal of unnecessary worry. More recently, the recall of the Dalkon Shield led many IUD users to seek advice and medical checks because they were not certain if this was the device they were wearing. The Dalkon Shield was recalled following allegations in America that it was associated with an increased incidence of infection among those who used it.

At one time it was possible to identify the IUD being worn by the colour of the threads attached to it (the doctor can normally see these threads on examination). This is no longer possible because some dyes are not used any more owing to possible health risks. If medical records are not available, the only way to check with certainty which device is being worn is to take it out! As IUD users are aware, the fitting and removal of an IUD is not something that should be treated so casually.

Being protected against unwanted pregnancy is a very important part of a woman's life. It is not fanciful to say that the ability to have the desired number of children, at times when this is planned, has been responsible for significant changes in the lives of millions of women. Because fertility regulation is so important, knowledge of the precise device being used is equally important. IUDs come in various models and sizes; be sure you know which model and size is being fitted, the 'life' of the device and the recommended frequency of follow-up visits.

Some doctors will take the time to demonstrate the IUD fitting with the use of a clear plastic model of the uterus. If asked, doctors will show the instruments to be used and explain their action, and offer reassurance about the sounds these instruments might make during use (for example, manipulation of the ratchet of a metal speculum creates a distinctive and potentially alarming sound). He or she will probably forewarn you that the fitting of the IUD and the examination which precedes it might cause some discomfort, but that this should quickly pass, and that some women experience slight bleeding and cramps during the first few days after fitting. The first few menstrual periods are also likely to be heavier and longer but this should gradually improve. The doctor will explain how to check the nylon threads of the IUD – these are attached to the bottom end of the device and pass through the cervical canal into the upper part of the vagina – every now and then. This gives reassurance that the device is indeed still in place in the uterus. The doctor will stress the need to seek medical advice should any untoward symptoms of pain or bleeding or vaginal discharge occur, or if a period is missed. A follow-up visit to make certain that the IUD is in good position and that no side effects have developed will be needed during the first three months.

The pelvic examination before IUD fitting

The dorsal position – where the woman lies on her back on the couch with knees bent and legs apart – is almost always used for pelvic examination. The actual fitting of the IUD, while normally performed in the dorsal position, is sometimes undertaken with the woman lying curled up on her left side (the left lateral position). Some doctors think that there is less embarrassment for the woman if she is lying on her side, but a recent survey showed that the majority of doctors have a strong preference for using the dorsal position. Among the reasons given for this preference were:

a) It is easier for the doctor to detect any abnormalities which may be present.
b) It is easier to communicate with the patient and judge her reactions better if there is face to face contact.
c) The patient can see what is going on and can communicate better with the doctor.
d) It is more comfortable for the doctor. Lighting facilities are usually designed for this position and instruments can be handled more efficiently (especially where the patient is at the end of the couch and the doctor is sitting down).
e) It is more comfortable for the patient.

The pelvic examination has two main purposes: first to check the size, shape and position of your uterus, and secondly to ensure that your reproductive organs are healthy. This will normally be accomplished in three stages:

i) an assessment using the hands only, called a **bimanual examination**;
ii) an examination using an instrument called a **speculum** which allows the doctor to see the vagina and cervix;
iii) the **sounding** of the uterus which entails the passing of a

slender straw-like instrument through the cervical canal to check for any obstruction and to measure the length of the uterus. The sound will also confirm the direction in which the uterus is lying which was previously noted at the bimanual examination.

Some doctors prefer to reverse the order of the first two phases and undertake the speculum examination first, to avoid the possibility of the bimanual examination disturbing the condition of the vagina and cervix. The disadvantage of this is that the speculum has to be removed for the bimanual examination and replaced again for IUD fitting. Some experienced doctors argue that this is unnecessarily disturbing for the woman being examined.

The bimanual examination

The doctor will first check that the external genital area appears healthy, before gently inserting his or her index and middle fingers into the vagina to examine the condition of the vagina and cervix. The doctor is feeling for any obstruction or roughness in the vagina or at the cervix. This examination will normally be painless.

The doctor's other hand will then be placed on the lower abdomen, and by gently pressing the abdomen it is possible to locate the uterus between the two hands. This will tell the doctor whether the uterus is lying in the anteverted, retroverted or mid-position.

The doctor is also feeling for the size and shape of the uterus. If it is larger than usual and is smooth and soft, a pregnancy might be suspected. If it is larger than usual and is irregular in shape, there may be fibroids present. Most women attending for an IUD fitting have neither of these conditions and the most the doctor will be doing is checking that all is well, and finding out just where the uterus is lying. The doctor will then feel the fallopian tubes and the ovaries, and ask if any pain is caused. During this internal examination there will be some mild discomfort as the uterus and its attachments are felt and gently moved, but any pain is abnormal and could indicate infection; it should be

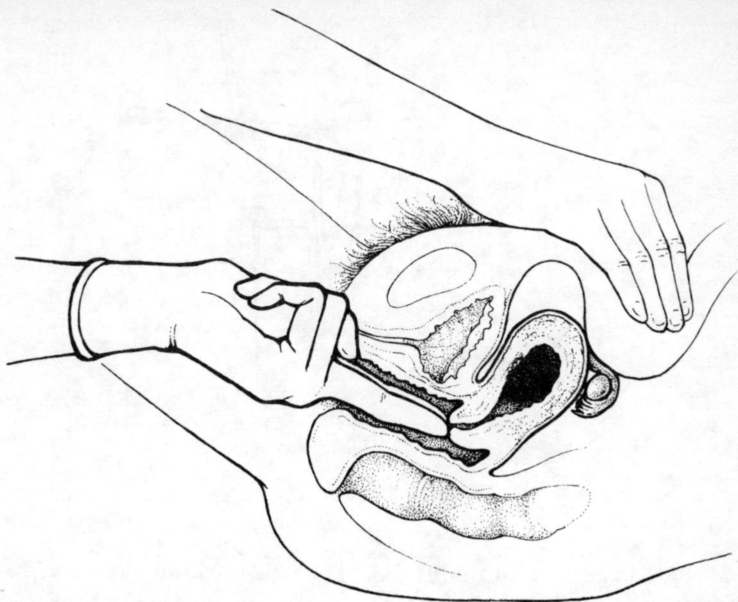

Figure 5 A bimanual examination to check the position, shape and size of the uterus

reported to the doctor. The bimanual examination should take only a few moments and is normally accomplished without undue trauma.

The speculum examination

The doctor will then fit a speculum into the vagina. This device is used to keep the walls of the vagina apart so that the doctor can see the vaginal walls and cervix clearly. It is made of either metal or plastic. The part which enters the vagina is the smooth, rounded part – there are no sharp edges – and although the speculum appears to be a large instrument, most of it remains outside the body. The speculum is gently inserted into the vagina in the closed position and then opened by means of a metal ratchet which holds the two blades in place; this can make quite a loud sound, but is no cause for alarm.

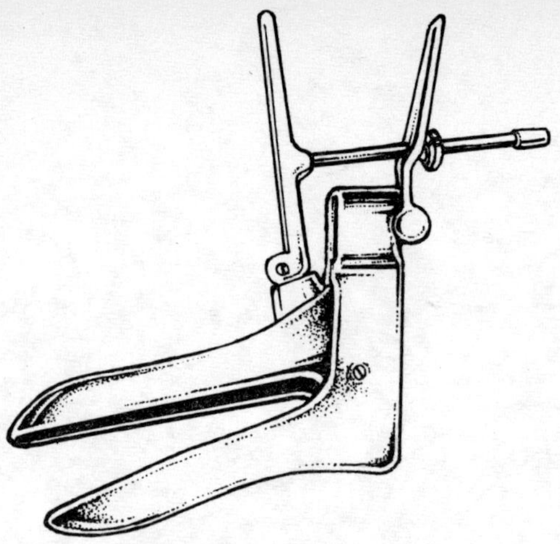

Figure 6a A speculum

Once the speculum is in place, the doctor will make a quick visual examination of the walls of the vagina and check the condition of the cervix. It is important to check that no infection is present. The two most common forms of vaginal infection are caused either by an organism called **trichomonas** or by a fungus called **monilia** (commonly called ' thrush'). Such infection would cause itching and inflammation of the vaginal walls and a discharge would be present (greenish-yellow and frothy in the case of trickomonas, and thick yellowish-white in the case of monilia). The cervix will normally be smooth, pink in colour, and

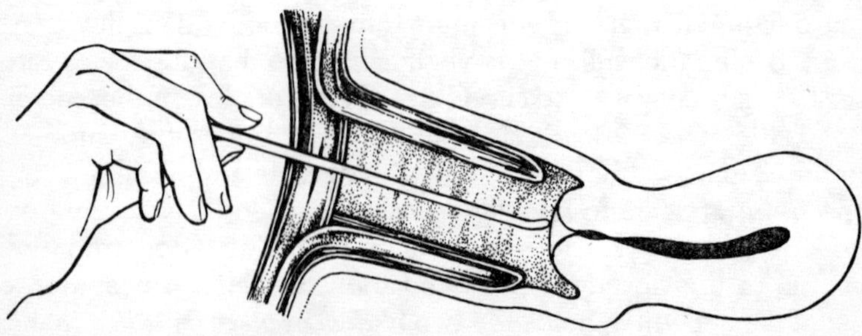

Figure 6b A cervical smear test

frequently a slight clear discharge may be present. These are all signs of a normal healthy cervix.

Occasionally, the cervix will show signs of an **erosion**. This condition is very common in women who have borne children. It is not a disease but merely describes a disturbance of the junction of the surface cells of the cervical canal and the cells of the cervix itself. After the stretching which occurs at child birth, the cervical canal cells sometimes spread over on to the surface of the cervix. This is usually nothing to worry about and the erosion often disappears spontaneously.

Rarely a cervical **polyp** may be found. This is a benign (i.e. non-malignant) growth which is simply a 'bunching up' of the lining cells of the cervix. Depending on its size and position it could interfere with IUD fitting. Polyps also tend to bleed easily if disturbed and treatment may be required before an IUD is fitted.

A routine cervical smear will also usually be taken. This procedure involves wiping a few cells from around the opening of the cervix on to a small wooden spatula. This can be felt, but it is not painful. Some doctors will also take this opportunity to collect any discharge from the cervix using a small cotton-wool swab. Both the cervical smear and the swab will be sent to the laboratory for testing. Any signs of abnormality will be reported to the doctor in due course, and if necessary appropriate remedial action taken.

Sounding of the uterus

Once the doctor is satisfied that all is well, the next step is usually to sound the uterus. There has been some discussion about the necessity for sounding in the medical literature in recent years, though most experienced family planning doctors accept that sounding should take place as it provides valuable information about the size and direction of the uterus and also reveals the very occasional uterine abnormality which would be a contra-indication to IUD fitting.

Before passing any instrument through the cervical canal, the doctor will clean the cervix using a sterile cotton-wool swab dipped in an antiseptic solution. The vagina is not sterile in the natural state, and therefore to attempt to create a completely sterile area would not be appropriate. But removal of vaginal secretions from the cervix will reduce the risk of any non-sterile material being pushed up into the uterus, an area which is normally germ-free.

There has also been much debate in recent years about the value of using an instrument to hold and steady the cervix at the time of sounding and IUD fitting. There are considerable advantages in the use of such an instrument, but it does sometimes cause a certain amount of discomfort. A single-toothed tenaculum is usually used to grasp the cervix; applied properly it should not be sharply painful, but it will result in a strong pinching sensation. Most women report this as unpleasant, but it is over very quickly and the discomfort does not persist.

The sound is a rounded slender instrument which passes through the cervical canal and into the uterus. Any obstruction resulting from previous scarring or from the presence of fibroids or other abnormality will be felt by the doctor. The length of the uterus can also be determined. The normal uterus measures about 65 mms from the opening of the cervix to its farthest point (the fundus). The sound passes out of the cervical canal and into the uterus through the internal os. At this time, some women experience a uterine spasm, which is most often described as a 'period-like cramping pain'. The most commonly used IUDs have inserters which are smaller than the sound and so once the sounding has taken place the worst is over. Some IUD users report that there was no discomfort experienced at sounding or IUD fitting.

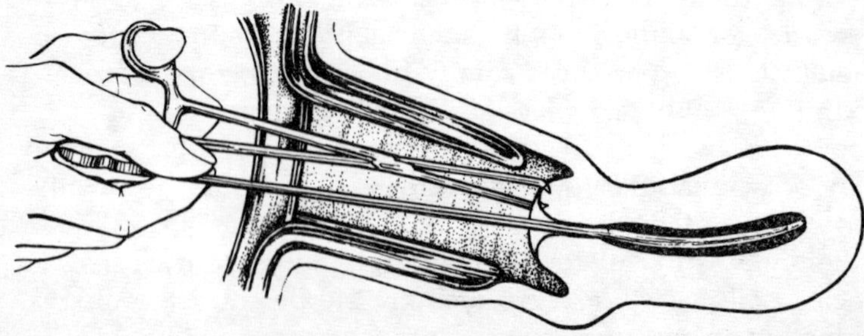

Figure 7 Sounding the uterus

Procedures and facilities do, of course, differ slightly from clinic to clinic and the examination procedures used by different doctors may vary in detail and not take place exactly as described here.

Fitting the IUD

An IUD fitting normally takes no more than three or four minutes. The position of the uterus and the type of IUD to be fitted will affect the detailed way in which the doctor will work, but the overall aim will be the same; to position the IUD correctly in the uterus as quickly and painlessly as possible. If a tenaculum has been used to hold the cervix during sounding, this will be left in place. It helps to straighten out the cervical canal and to line it up with the direction of the uterus. The tenaculum also provides counter-traction when the IUD and inserter are eased through the cervical canal. The doctor will again clean the cervix using a mild antiseptic solution.

Different IUD models require slightly different techniques for insertion into the uterus. The four most commonly used IUDs show the differing techniques in IUD fitting very clearly. The Multiload IUD rests on the end of a hollow tube with only the stem of the device in the tube; the IUD and tube are gently passed through the cervical canal, and once correctly placed in the uterus the inserter is gently withdrawn leaving the IUD in the uterus. Other devices are folded inside the hollow inserter tube. Once in the uterus an inner rod is used either to push out the IUD from the inserter tube or to hold the IUD steady while the outer inserter tube is withdrawn backwards over the IUD. The first technique (called the push-in technique by doctors) is usually associated with the Lippes Loop and the second (the 'withdrawal' technique) with the Gravigard and Novagard devices, but either technique can be used with any device. Other devices may have aids to assist the loading of the IUD into the inserter tube but these are small variations of the above techniques and are clearly explained on the IUD packaging. Devices are normally loaded into the inserter tube just before fitting; this ensures that when they are released into the uterus they will quickly resume their original shape. If they are left too

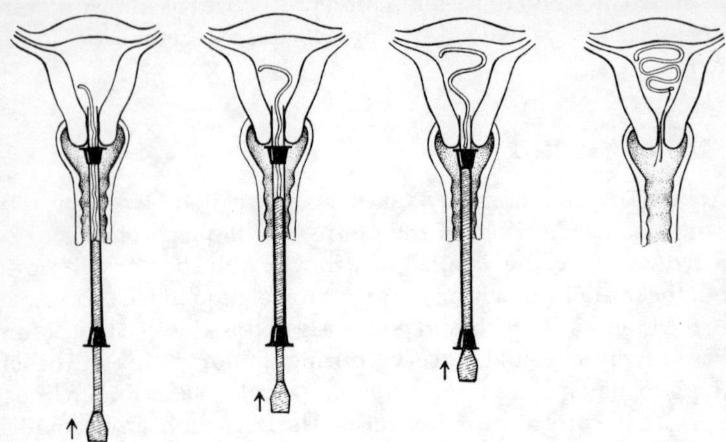

Figure 8a The 'push-in' technique

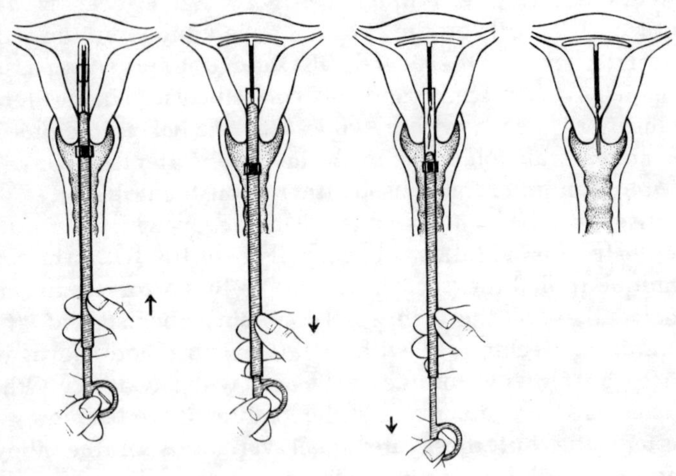

Figure 8b The 'withdrawal' technique

long in the inserter tube, their shape may become distorted and they may fail to unfold properly when released into the uterus.

After the inserter tube has been removed, the threads of the IUD will be left protruding from the cervix and lying in the vagina. Once satisfied that the IUD is correctly placed, the doctor will cut the threads at about 2.5 cm from the external os. The tenaculum and the speculum will be gently removed. Sometimes there is slight bleeding where the tenaculum has held the cervix, but this usually stops quickly (sanitary protection will be provided if necessary). You will then be encouraged to sit up and rest for a few moments.

How to feel for the IUD threads

After the IUD has been fitted you will be told how to check that the device is still in position by feeling for the threads attached to it. Most IUDs have two threads about the same thickness as button thread and generally made of nylon. These also facilitate removal of the IUD. When the time comes to remove the IUD, this can be done easily by pulling gently on the threads. The material from which the threads are made should not deteriorate or disintegrate and so they can be used over a considerable length of time.

If the threads have been cut to the correct length, they should not be felt by your partner during sexual intercourse. There have been isolated reports of men complaining that they can feel the sharp cut end of the threads. If this happens, you should return to the clinic so the doctor can trim the threads for you.

Women are often advised to feel for the threads after each menstrual period. This is intended to reassure the woman that the IUD is still in place and that all is well. However, it is thought that very few IUD users follow this advice and the IUD threads often remain unfelt for months at a time, if not for the whole period the IUD is being worn. Despite reassurances at the time of fitting that feeling for the threads is a comparatively easy procedure, many IUD users do not appear to find it so. The threads are fine and tend to be slippery, partly due to the nylon material used in their manufacture, but also because of the presence of vaginal mucus. As the threads cannot be seen, and the woman is often balancing on one foot, it is not surprising that many give up the attempt. On follow-up visits the examining doctor will check visually for the presence of the threads.

IUD follow-up visits

You should make an appointment for a follow-up visit to check all is well before leaving the clinic after the IUD has been fitted. For most women the follow-up examination is similar to that before IUD fitting, but it does not usually involve passing a sound into the uterus. An internal examination usually takes place and, providing all is well, this requires the use of a speculum only. The doctor may also take the opportunity to do a cervical smear test which, although having no direct connection with IUD use, is part of the general health care being provided.

Before leaving the clinic after the IUD has been fitted or after a follow-up visit, you should be sure you have the following information:

i) the name and size (where applicable) of the IUD model being worn;
ii) the length of time before the IUD requires routine re-fitting;
iii) the date when the next follow-up visit is due, and how this is to be arranged;
iv) the procedures to be followed if additional advice about any aspect of IUD use is required. This will require details of when telephone contact can be made and to whom any enquiry should be made.

If the doctor or clinic does not supply this information on a prepared card, make a record of it yourself and keep it in a safe place.

Questions sometimes asked by women attending for an IUD fitting

What is the risk of my becoming pregnant?

On average between 1 and 2 in every 100 IUD users will become pregnant in any one year. There is some variation in this number depending upon the type of IUD model fitted and the fertility of the woman using the IUD (more detailed figures are given in Chapter 7). Discounting male and female sterilisation which are permanent methods of contraception, the IUD is second in effectiveness to the pill. The risk of becoming pregnant when using no contraceptive method at all when engaging in a regular sexual relationship is up to thirty times higher (see Chapter 1 for a comparative assessment of the different methods).

How does the IUD work?

The short answer to this question is that no one is quite sure. Most researchers accept that one or more of the following mechanisms are probably involved:

a) the IUD acts as a foreign body and stimulates an inflammatory reaction in the uterus. This causes the production of very large numbers of cells called *macrophages* which appear in the fluids present in the uterus. The function of these cells is to ingest any foreign material and it is suggested that any sperm (or a fertilised ovum) which may arrive in the uterus are consumed by these excessively large number of macrophages;

b) the presence of an IUD may increase the activity of the fallopian tubes and may cause the ovum to pass along the tube quicker than usual. The ovum normally goes through a process of maturation or ripening as it passes along the fallopian tube on its journey from the ovary to the uterus, and fertilisation usually takes place in the tube. If the journey along the tube is speeded up, the ovum may not be sufficiently mature for fertilisation to take place;

c) the inflammatory changes in the lining of the uterus which are provoked by the IUD may prevent a fertilised egg from implanting in the uterine wall and so stop it progressing on to its next stage of development;

d) copper IUDs release copper ions into the uterus, and these may alter the composition or consistency of the mucus in the cervical canal. This change in consistency may prevent sperm from penetrating the mucus.

e) IUDs which release hormones may also prevent ovulation.

From this list it can be seen that a number of different actions may be taking place, but the precise influence of each is still not known at the present time.

For how long will the IUD be effective?

Most IUDs can be left in place for several years, and will continue to prevent pregnancy without harmful effect until they are removed. Some inert plastic IUDs can be left in place indefinitely; ten years or more is not unusual. Other devices which contain copper require replacement after a stipulated interval, usually two to five years. No IUD in regular use needs routine replacement in less than two years. Only one infrequently fitted hormone-releasing IUD – the Progestasert – has to be replaced after a shorter interval.

How soon can I have intercourse without taking other precautions?

The IUD gives protection against pregnancy immediately it is fitted.

Should I take special precautions in the first few weeks after fitting, until the IUD settles?

This is not strictly necessary. It is known that the IUD is more likely to be expelled from the uterus during the first month or two after fitting than at any other time. This is one reason why an early check-up is necessary. It is advisable to check for the presence of the IUD regularly during these first few weeks.

How do I know if the IUD is in place?

The threads which are attached to the IUD can be felt in the vagina. Pain during intercourse or slight bleeding after intercourse may indicate that the IUD has partially expelled into the cervical canal, and this should be reported to your doctor immediately.

Can I still use tampons?

Yes. There is no reason why tampons should not continue to be used after IUD fitting. Very occasionally an IUD is dislodged when a tampon is removed, but this is probably due to the IUD being already expelled into the vagina and not to the use of the tampon.

Will the IUD fitting hurt?

There is some discomfort associated with an IUD fitting. Most women say it is no worse than a sharp period pain and that the discomfort does not last for long. One of the instruments used (a tenaculum) may cause a sharp pinching sensation, but this is very transient. When asked to compare the discomfort of IUD fitting with the discomfort of going to the dentist, most women thought IUD fitting was no more uncomfortable.

Will I be able to have a baby as soon as I have stopped using the IUD?

It is estimated that about one-third of all women wishing to conceive after IUD removal do so within one month. This proportion rises to over 7 out of 10 within a year, and over 9 out of 10 within two years. These figures relate to women who have already had at least one baby sometime in the past and have therefore demonstrated their fertility. The proportions will be lower for women of unproven fertility, or who are over the age of 35 years.

If I become pregnant when wearing the IUD will the baby be harmed in any way?

In the unlikely event of a pregnancy, and if the woman wishes to continue with her pregnancy, there is about a 50/50 chance that the pregnancy will end in a miscarriage. In any pregnancy there is a slight chance that the baby will be born with a handicap or deformity. There is no evidence that the IUD causes any abnormality, and if the pregnancy goes to term, the chances of having a completely normal baby are as good for the mother wearing an IUD as for a mother who is not wearing an IUD.

If I do become pregnant, will I be allowed to have an abortion?

The same rules governing abortion apply to IUD users as to any other women experiencing an unwanted pregnancy. The use of a contraceptive method which has failed is evidence that an unplanned pregnancy may have disadvantages to the mother, the child or to other members of the family. This type of evidence is assessed when considering whether or not to approve an abortion. It should be remembered that the unplanned pregnancy rate is very low, and the question of whether or not to request an abortion has to be considered by very few IUD users. Any IUD user who misses a menstrual period or who otherwise suspects a pregnancy should seek medical advice straight away.

Will the IUD affect my periods?

Women often find that their periods are heavier and sometimes slightly longer than those they experienced before having the IUD fitted. This problem, when it occurs, often settles after a few months. Nevertheless complaints of disturbance to the menstrual cycle are the major reasons for IUD removal. Even so this affects an average of less than 1 in 10 of all IUD users; the precise figure depends on the IUD being used, the age and parity of the woman, and the correct placing of the IUD in the uterus. Occasionally the IUD causes slight intermittent bleeding or 'spotting' between periods. Hormone-releasing IUDs appear to have a higher risk of this type of bleeding than other IUDs.

How often will I need to come back for check-ups?

The usual practice is for a follow-up visit to be suggested about six weeks after the IUD fitting (i.e. after the next menstrual period). Subsequent routine follow-up visits are usually arranged for the yearly anniversary of the IUD fitting. If an IUD of a relatively new kind is being fitted, more frequent follow-up checks may be requested.

Does the IUD cause pelvic infection?

IUD use is associated with a small increase in the likelihood of pelvic infection, but most researchers would argue that the IUD does not actually *cause* infection. Other forms of contraception (e.g. the pill, the cap and the condom) help to *prevent* infection but the IUD does not. In fact, because it acts as a foreign body the IUD will aggravate any infection that does occur. Other factors can contribute to the incidence of infection, particularly the number of sexual partners a woman has (and the number of sexual partners that partner has). Recent figures obtained from a study which compared the experience of over 13,000 IUD users has shown that the incidence of infection among these British women is about one case among every 100 IUD users each year, irrespective of the IUD model being worn.

What should I do if the IUD is expelled?

If the IUD comes out it is important to make an appointment to see the doctor as soon as possible. If intercourse has recently taken place, and it is in the fertile period during the middle of the menstrual cycle, conception could occur because sperm can live for up to three or four days in the reproductive tract.

Another form of contraception should be used temporarily. It is possible that a different type of IUD model, or a larger sized device could be fitted and remain in place quite satisfactorily.

Does the clinic inform my own doctor about the fitting?

It is important for the family doctor to know about any medical treatment which his patients may have received elsewhere, and the clinic doctor will routinely communicate with the GP. If for any particular reason you do not wish your family doctor to be told, the clinic doctor will respect your wishes in this matter.

If I move to another area how can I arrange follow-up visits?

It is advisable to contact the clinic before moving so that you can be given details of your IUD to pass on to your new medical advisor. The clinic may also be able to give you addresses of family planning clinics in your new area.

How much will the IUD fitting and follow-up cost?

In the UK this service is provided free of charge under the national health service (NHS). If you, or the fitting doctor, prefer to use an IUD which is one not normally provided under the NHS, the device (but not the doctor's time) will have to be paid for. Devices are not expensive. Most family planning clinics provide devices which have been purchased by the local health authority. If you decide to have an IUD fitted privately it is wise to ask for a statement of costs for both IUD fitting and follow-up, *in advance of the fitting*. Be sure also to find out the recommended frequency of follow-up visits and how often the IUD should be removed and replaced. This will give an indication of the total cost involved.

Will the IUD affect my sex life?

The wearing of an IUD may make sexual activity more spontaneous, partly because there is no need to remember to make contraceptive preparations, and partly because the removal of the fear of pregnancy may make sexual activity more enjoyable. On the other hand, the increased duration of menstrual bleeding often associated with IUD use may reduce the opportunity for sexual intercourse.

As far as the sex act itself is concerned, some IUD users worry that their partner may be able to feel the IUD in place. There have been occasional reports of male discomfort, mainly associated with the nylon threads which are attached to the device. This is usually resolved by a second trimming of the threads at a subsequent follow-up check visit.

Does the IUD cause cancer?

There is no evidence whatsoever that wearing an IUD increases the risk of cancer.

Do I need my husband's consent to have an IUD fitted?

This may seem a chauvinistic question to ask in the 1980s, but as recently as ten years ago it was commonly assumed that a husband's consent was necessary. In 1977, the National Council for Civil Liberties challenged the requirement of one area health authority that a woman needed her husband's consent for the fitting of an IUD. The health authority changed its policy after legal advice that there was no justification for such a requirement and that those who demanded it could be considered to be in breach of the sex discrimination laws.

Most husbands who have volunteered information about the use of an IUD by their wives have indicated that they wish to offer support to their wives, but that they are uncertain about how to go about this. A feeling of exclusion is often reported; 'it's women's business' is the comment most frequently made. Yet there is a desire to offer support even if this is confined to providing transport and reading a newspaper in the car parked outside during (sometimes lengthy) clinic visits.

Even though the question of consent does not arise, it is still very important to discuss the use of any contraceptive method with your partner. The most successful IUD users appear to be those who have come to a considered and well-informed decision about IUD use; a full consideration can only be undertaken if the subject is viewed from the perspective of both partners. Unhappily there may be some women who read this who do not have an understanding and supportive partner, and who believe that the use of other contraceptive methods may be disruptive or otherwise unsuitable. Apart from sterilisation, the IUD is the only contraceptive method which does not require daily or periodic use, with the attendant need for storing supplies. It is possible to be a discreet IUD user if this is necessary.

CHAPTER 5

Possible side effects

Once a woman has opted to use an IUD for contraceptive purposes and has had the device fitted, there are four possible outcomes:

i) she continues to wear the IUD without any complaint or difficulty;
ii) the IUD is removed for reasons which may or may not be directly related to the IUD;
iii) the IUD is expelled from the uterus;
iv) she becomes pregnant while wearing the IUD.

These outcomes or 'events' have been listed in the order in which they most commonly occur. It should be stressed that only a relatively small number of women require removal of the device or experience an expulsion or pregnancy. On the other hand women in the first category of satisfied IUD users account for 80-90 per cent of all women who are fitted with an IUD each year. So the following description of some of the possible side effects of IUD use will be relevant to only a small minority of all the women who use the IUD as a means of contraception.

For those of us involved in research into IUD use, there is a fifth category of IUD users to consider: those women who can no longer be contacted in order to determine how they are faring with the IUD. For a variety of reasons, IUD users sometimes fail to attend for follow-up visits. The numbers in this category are important for the interpretation of the statistics being collected. If a high proportion of women become 'lost to follow-up' the validity of published rates for removal, expulsion and pregnancy for those women who are not 'lost' will be suspect. The experience of the women who do not return for check-ups may be different from the experience of those who do. It is for this reason that published reports about IUD results should be assessed carefully. Not only do the characteristics of the woman wearing the device and of the doctor fitting the device affect the outcome of IUD use; the design and conduct of the research study must also be meticulously correct if the results are to be believed.

When the IUD has to be removed

Removal of the IUD is usually a simple and virtually painless procedure. The threads are grasped with a pair of forceps, and gentle pulling is usually sufficient to draw out the device from the uterus. Sometimes a spasm of the uterine muscle may occur as the device passes through the internal os, and this may cause a cramping period-like pain. Occasionally the threads disappear from the vagina because they have been drawn up into the uterus, perhaps by movement of the device. In these cases the doctor can often bring down the threads using a thin flexible plastic instrument known as a thread retriever. In rare cases, if the threads cannot be found or if the device has become distorted, a woman may need referral to a gynaecologist to have the device removed.

Some common reasons for IUD removal do not imply dissatisfaction but, on the contrary, reflect satisfactory use of the device. For instance a device may have reached the end of its useful life and may require routine removal and re-fitting. With copper devices this is usually recommended after two or five years, but inert plastic devices may also require routine removal, if they have become encrusted with a deposit after several years. Alternatively, a woman who has been satisfied with her IUD may wish to have the device removed because she now wishes to have another baby.

An IUD should also be removed when a woman has reached the menopause and no longer needs contraceptive protection. This is usually done when periods have completely ceased for about a year. It is not thought advisable to leave the IUD in place after the menopause, as the more fragile lining of the uterus may be irritated by the device.

In addition to these common reasons for IUD removal, there is a further category which is not directly related to the IUD itself, but which reflects the changing medical or personal needs of the woman wearing the IUD. This group includes removal of the IUD to facilitate the treatment of a medical problem which, while having nothing directly to do with the IUD, is made more difficult if the IUD is left in place. (The treatment of a gynaecological disorder is an obvious example.) Alternatively either the woman or her husband may decide that they definitely want no more children, and one of the partners may undergo sterilisation. In this case the IUD will no longer be required.

Separating off these reasons from the more negative medical reasons directly linked to IUD use is important. Successful IUD use is seldom emphasised in the publicity given to IUDs. This is not to argue that medical complaints should be ignored or underestimated, but merely to point out that successful IUD use is the normal experience of most women.

Possible side effects of IUD use

However, sometimes removal of the IUD is necessary because of dissatisfaction with the device and because of unpleasant side effects associated with its use.

Bleeding and/or pain

The most common unpleasant side effect associated with IUD use is increased blood loss at menstruation. This is sometimes accompanied with cramp-like period pain. Most women will have been warned to expect heavier periods for the first few months after having an IUD fitted. The assumption is that these heavier periods eventually settle back to normal, but research evidence does not support this theory. Reports that periods become lighter again may have more to do with the women becoming resigned to the increase over time and therefore complaining less about it, rather than to any actual decrease in blood loss. What objective evidence there is suggests that increased levels are maintained for a considerable time.

The type of IUD model worn appears to determine to some extent the amount of increased blood loss, but the woman's age and previous child-bearing experience are also important. Periods do often become heavier once a woman has given birth to children, and sometimes as a woman becomes older she also finds that her periods are heavier. Research studies which have measured actual amounts of menstrual loss experienced by women over a period of time suggest that if one of the larger inert plastic IUDs is worn (e.g. the Lippes Loop or the Saf-T-Coil) menstrual loss is increased to about twice the normal amount. The smaller, more flexible, copper-carrying devices are associated with a smaller increase, but a rough estimate of one and a half times as much blood loss is often given. An added problem is that quite often this increase in the *amount* of blood loss is also accompanied by an increase in the *duration* of blood loss; this is particularly so with the copper-carrying IUDs. So not only may periods be heavier, they may also be longer. However, it is important to remember that all women are different and that the amount of 'normal' menstrual loss varies widely from woman to woman. Some women normally have light, non-painful periods; other women may, from the time they first start to menstruate, always have quite heavy and perhaps painful periods. In each case this is normal for them. If, after IUD fitting, the woman who normally has light periods finds that her loss has increased to twice the amount, this amount of loss may still be acceptable and not too inconvenient. But the same increase is likely to be much more of a problem to the woman who started off from a baseline of relatively heavy periods in the first place.

The precise reasons why an IUD causes increased levels of blood loss are not properly understood. It probably has something to do with disturbance of blood vessels in the soft lining of the uterus, or to an alteration in the normal clotting mechanism of the blood. It is known that the fitting of an IUD is associated with an increase in the presence of certain enzymes which, among other biochemical effects, also affect blood clotting.

Besides the increase in both duration and amount of blood loss, women wearing an IUD may also experience shorter menstrual cycles with the period starting rather earlier than usual. This has led some researchers to conclude that the presence of an IUD makes the uterus less responsive to the action of progesterone, one of the key hormones influencing the progress of each menstrual cycle.

The new focus in IUD research is the development of hormone-releasing IUDs which will prevent this increase in blood loss. The most well known of these is the Progestasert IUD which each day releases 65 micrograms of the hormone progesterone directly into the uterus. But while this device has successfully achieved a reduction in the *amount* of blood lost, it tends to increase the *frequency* of blood loss; and the time when this loss is likely to occur is no longer predictable. As progesterone taken in the form of oral contraception or by injection is also related to disturbance of the menstrual cycle, it is not surprising that this occurs when the hormone is released directly into the uterus itself.

A considerable amount of work is being carried out on testing various other compounds which could be released into the uterus, but progress is slow and sometimes disheartening. The long-term effects of drugs taken into the body by this route are also unknown and therefore great care has to be taken in their development and use. Some progress is being made though, and the next drug-releasing IUD to be made generally available is one which releases the drug 'levonorgestrel' directly in the uterus. It is hoped that this device will reduce both the amount of menstrual loss and the occurrence of menstrual pain. Its success however will depend upon its ability not only to control the amount of menstrual loss, but also the duration, frequency and predictability of that loss, whilst at the same time maintaining a high degree of protection against pregnancy. While the more traditional IUDs may be found wanting in relation to the increased amount of blood loss, it is usually possible to predict fairly accurately when bleeding is likely to occur. A recent World Health Organisation research study showed that women are more disturbed by menstrual blood loss being unpredictable than they are by periods being heavy. However, increased menstrual blood loss may lead to iron-deficiency anaemia, though research into iron levels among IUD users remains inconclusive; while some studies have found a reduction, others have not. A large-scale American study undertaken in 1981 showed that women wearing an IUD were at no greater risk of anaemia than women not wearing an IUD.

Treatment for increased menstrual bleeding and/or pain when wearing an IUD

It may be possible to control painful periods by taking one of the usual analgesic drugs. However, some doctors advise that those preparations which contain aspirin should not be used. This is because aspirin is believed to reduce the biochemical response of the uterus to the IUD, so leading to a reduction in the ability of the IUD to protect against pregnancy. Drugs are also available which will reduce the amount of menstrual bleeding if this is considered to be excessive, but again the use of some of these drugs may have a similar effect to aspirin. If pain or increased bleeding is persistent, an examination may be required to determine its cause, and a recommendation may be made for the IUD to be removed.

Table 1 shows that the removal of an IUD because of bleeding or pain varies according to the device used and the age and parity of the woman. Only the IUDs in common use at the present time are included in the table. On average about 10 in every 100 IUD users will have their IUD removed for this reason within one year of fitting. The figures have been obtained from over 25,000 IUD users attending one of the forty-six family planning clinics taking part in the UK IUD Research Network.

Infection

A careful assessment of the experience of over 10,000 IUD wearers in the United Kingdom has shown that between 1 and 2 women in every 100 will need to have their IUD removed because of an infection known as 'pelvic inflammatory disease' or PID. Despite the small number of women who experience PID it is regarded as a serious condition, not only because of its immediate debilitating effects, but also because of its known relationship with subfertility. Pelvic infection can cause damage and scarring to the delicate lining of the fallopian tube. This damage makes it difficult or even impossible for the mature ovum to pass along the fallopian tube to the uterus, thereby also making conception difficult or impossible.

It is generally recognised that the use of an IUD exposes the

Table 1 Removal of IUD following a complaint of bleeding and/or pain during the first year

Type of IUD User	Gravigard (Cu 7)	Gyne T (Cu T)	Novagard	Multiload	Saf-T-Coil	Lippes Loop C	Lippes Loop D
No previous birth	Moderate* (7.9)	Moderate (8.4)	Moderate (6.5)	High (10.8)	**	**	**
1 or 2 previous births	Moderate (8.9)	Moderate (6.5)	Low (4.4)	Moderate (9.0)	High (12.9)	High (10.5)	Moderate (8.5)
3 or more previous births	Moderate (8.3)	Low (4.9)	Moderate (6.2)	High (11.3)	High (11.3)	Moderate (8.5)	Moderate (9.0)
Under 30 years with 1 or 2 previous births	Moderate (9.1)	Moderate (6.6)	Moderate (5.5)	Moderate (9.6)	High (12.0)	High (13.1)	Moderate (9.6)
30 and over with 1 or 2 previous births	Moderate (8.6)	Moderate (6.3)	Low (4.0)	Moderate (8.2)	High (14.8)	High (12.1)	High (11.8)

Numbers in brackets give the risk for every 100 IUD users during the first year of use
* For definition of 'high', 'moderate' and 'low', see page 00
** Insufficient fittings

woman to an increased risk of infection of the reproductive organs. Of all the side effects of IUD use, PID has attracted more publicity in recent years than any other complication. This is mostly due to the publicity given to one particular IUD – the Dalkon Shield – whose users were alleged to be particularly vulnerable to this problem. If pelvic infection is associated with subsequent infertility, and the IUD is associated with pelvic infection, then the argument that IUDs should not be worn by women who might wish to have a baby in the future has considerable force.

However like most associations described in a rather oversimplified way, the reality is more complicated. While accepting that the *risk* of infection is increased among IUD users, a number of studies have shown that the *experience* of such infection is no worse among some IUD users than it is among other women who are using a different form of contraception or no contraceptive method at all. This apparent contradiction is due to the presence of other factors which may be influencing the likelihood of infection in ways that the IUD cannot prevent. While most researchers agree that there is a raised risk of pelvic infection among IUD users, many disagree about why this should be so. Some claim that placing an IUD in a previously sterile uterus after introducing it through a non-sterile vagina is a sure way to introduce infection. Others point to the ability of bacteria to enter the uterus by means of the threads attached to the IUD at one end, and with the other end lying in the vagina. (It was this theory which was used to explain the alleged high incidence of infection among Dalkon Shield users.) Other research has shown that the reported infection was unlikely to have been introduced in this way and that other causes must be sought. The risk of PID appears to vary widely, depending on the health, ability to resist disease, and the number and frequency of sexual contacts of those concerned. While the IUD may not cause PID, unlike barrier contraceptive methods and some oral contraceptives it cannot prevent the occurrence of infection. Hormone-releasing IUDs are being developed which may directly combat PID, but these are not yet generally available.

Symptoms which may cause a woman to suspect she has a pelvic infection include abnormal vaginal discharge, heavy bleeding and lower abdominal pain and tenderness. The woman may also feel generally unwell and may run a temperature. It is important that a doctor should be consulted as soon as possible so that treatment can be commenced and the infection prevented from spreading more widely and becoming more severe. In relatively mild cases treatment with antibiotics may be sufficient to clear up the infection and it may not be necessary to remove the IUD. Removal of the IUD will become necessary if the infection is severe.

Expulsion of the IUD

The type of IUD model being worn, the shape, size and muscular tone of the uterus, and the technique of the doctor who fitted the IUD all affect the incidence of IUD expulsion. The likelihood of a device being expelled depends on how closely the shape and size of the device 'fits' the shape and size of the individual uterus into which it is fitted, as well as to the extent to which the device is able to absorb normal uterine contractions.

The risk of IUD expulsion is highest in the first month after fitting and this risk declines rapidly as each month passes. This is one of the reasons why an early follow-up visit is advised. The reduction in the risk of expulsion over time is quite dramatic. Very few expulsions occur after the first year of use; it has been estimated that the risk of expulsion during the third year of IUD use is about thirty-five times less than the risk of an expulsion occurring within the first three months of IUD fitting. This higher risk of expulsion immediately after IUD fitting applies even when one IUD is removed and a new one refitted immediately. Whilst not reaching the same level as after a first fitting, an increased risk is nevertheless present at each IUD refitting.

Because of the changes which take place in the size and shape of the uterus, women who have had a baby within the previous three months should be extra vigilant about possible IUD expulsion. There is also a higher risk of expulsion among women who have not yet had a baby, and among women under the age of 30 years. The firmer muscle tone of the uterus in younger, nulliparous women is likely to be related to this increased risk of expulsion.

Table 2 Risk of IUD expulsion during the first year

Type of IUD User	Gravigard (Cu 7)	Gyne T (Cu T)	Novagard	Multiload	Saf-T-Coil	Lippes Loop C	Lippes Loop D
No previous birth	High* (11.1)	Moderate (9.3)	Very low (0.0)	Moderate (6.1)	**	**	**
1 or 2 previous births	High (10.0)	Moderate (5.5)	Low (3.9)	Moderate (5.4)	Moderate (9.7)	Moderate (7.1)	Moderate (6.0)
3 or more previous births	Moderate (6.0)	Low (3.3)	Low (4.6)	Very low (1.7)	Moderate (6.4)	Low (3.6)	Low (4.4)
Under 30 years with 1 or 2 previous births	High (11.4)	Moderate (7.2)	Moderate (8.2)	Moderate (6.6)	High (10.4)	High (10.3)	Moderate (6.5)
30 and over with 1 or 2 previous births	Moderate (6.1)	Very low (2.6)	Very low (2.0)	Low (3.5)	Moderate (8.0)	Low (4.7)	Low (3.5)

Numbers in brackets give the risk for every 100 IUD users during the first year of use
* For definition of 'high', 'moderate' and 'low', see page 00
** Insufficient fittings

Some IUDs have been specifically designed to resist expulsion. These 'fundal-seeking' IUDs may have attachments to the body of the device which help to push it further to the top (or fundus) of the uterus each time a contraction of the uterine muscle takes place. It should be noted that muscular contractions of the uterus are not confined to the time a child is being born; they occur in the non-pregnant uterus also, although at a much reduced strength. Size for size the uterus is probably the most powerful organ of the body and it is not surprising that an IUD is sometimes expelled. Other types of IUD are designed to resist these uterine contractions by changing and adapting their shape to absorb the contractions as they occur. It is also believed that copper or hormone-releasing IUDs have a quieting action on the uterine muscle which makes expulsion of the device less likely. A device which incorporates fundal-seeking characteristics, is flexible in the presence of uterine contractions, and carries copper or a progestogen-based hormone would then be expected to have a very low expulsion rate, and this has been demonstrated to be so. The Multiload and Novagard are such devices and reference to Table 2 will confirm the low expulsion rates. But, alas, a reduction in IUD expulsion is also often accompanied by an increase in complaints of bleeding or pain. It seems that if the uterus cannot expel the IUD an increased level of menstrual discomfort is likely. By contrast, devices which have a high risk of expulsion tend to be associated with lower levels of menstrual disturbance. Research into hormone-releasing IUDs continues in the hope that devices can be found which will both reduce expulsion and control blood loss, but as yet these are not generally available.

Most women notice if their IUD has been expelled and so are aware that they are no longer protected against pregnancy. Should this happen an alternative form of contraception must be used and an appointment made to see the doctor as soon as possible. If the IUD has been expelled at the fertile time of the menstrual cycle, and intercourse has recently taken place, conception could occur because sperm can live for up to three or four days in the female reproductive tract. After an expulsion it is often possible for the doctor to re-fit a slightly larger device, or a device which is known to be particularly resistant to expulsion.

Less frequently, expulsions take place without the woman's knowledge, usually at the time of menstruation when the IUD is removed from the vagina together with a tampon or, more rarely, when the woman is constipated. Sometimes the IUD is only partially expelled from the uterus and is found lying partly in the cervical canal by the doctor undertaking a follow-up examination. In such cases the IUD will be removed and replaced with another. Sometimes, a device which has partially expelled may be the cause of intermittent, slight bleeding or may cause pain during intercourse. If these symptoms occur they should be reported to a doctor so that the position of the IUD can be checked.

Both complete and partial expulsions are included in the expulsion rates given in Table 2. Some devices, if they expel, tend to be completely expelled from the uterus (e.g. the Multiload). Other devices (e.g. the Gravigard) are more prone to partial expulsion which is less likely to be noticed by the woman. This suggests that regular checking for the presence of the IUD by feeling for the threads, and conscientious attendance for follow-up visits are very important. A good idea is to check for the threads at the end of each menstrual period, as then you can be reassured that even if the threads are missing, you are definitely not pregnant, and you can use an alternative contraceptive method until you have arranged for a check-up.

Unintentional pregnancy

The risk of becoming unintentionally pregnant when wearing an IUD is, on average, between 1 and 2 in every 100 women during the first year of use. There is a slow but steady decline in this rate for subsequent years. This means that out of every 100 women who start wearing an IUD, up to 2 will have experienced a pregnancy before they have completed wearing the IUD for a whole year. It is not possible to be more precise than this because so much depends on factors not directly related to the IUD itself, but to the person wearing the IUD and to the person fitting the IUD. The important characteristics relating to the woman using the IUD include her age, the frequency and timing of sexual intercourse, and whether or not she has previously had a baby.

With increasing age, a woman's natural fertility declines and this will be reflected in the pregnancy rates reported. The number of previous pregnancies also gives some indication of a woman's fertility; some women are more fertile and tend to get pregnant more easily than other women. The interaction between a woman's age, parity and exposure to pregnancy has a marked effect upon reported pregnancy rates.

The factors associated with the person fitting the IUD were discussed in Chapter 4, but it is worth recalling that the skill of the person fitting the IUD is probably as important as the IUD model itself. The correct positioning of the IUD in the fundus of the uterus is necessary if efficient use is to be obtained. The doctor who is manually dexterous, and confident and well practised, will increase the efficiency of the IUD in preventing pregnancy.

None of this should suggest that the IUD model itself is of no consequence. Of course the shape, size and composition of the IUD are important, but it is a mistake to consider the intrinsic characteristics of the IUD model in isolation from these other factors. Bearing in mind the limitations of the figures presented, the pregnancy rates for different IUD models are summarised in Table 3. A comparison between the rate of unintentional pregnancy among IUD users and users of other methods of contraception is given in Chapter 2.

The pregnancy rate among IUD users tends to decline over time; this means that the small chance of becoming pregnant is reduced even further during the second year, and is still less in the third year, and so on. Reference to the low risk of pregnancy is of little comfort to those who do become unintentionally pregnant; but whilst some do become pregnant, the vast majority do not. Rumours of unwanted pregnancies can serve to create uncertainty about the efficiency of the IUD. In one study completed in the mid-1970s, a survey was undertaken in which questions were asked about unwanted pregnancies among IUD users. The total rumoured figure was in excess of seven times the figure recorded at the family planning clinic. Even after allowing for possible inaccuracy and duplication, the difference between the two sets of figures is remarkable. One thing is certain; the chance of an unwanted pregnancy occurring is small and likely to

Table 3 Risk of unplanned pregnancy during the first year

Type of IUD User	Gravigard (Cu 7)	Gyne T (Cu T)	Novagard	Multiload	Saf-T-Coil	Lippes Loop C	Lippes Loop D
No previous birth	Low (1.2)	Very low (0.9)	Moderate (2.2)	Very low (0.0)	**	**	**
1 or 2 previous births	Low (1.7)	Very low (0.9)	Very low (0.0)	Low (1.5)	Low (1.4)	Low (1.0)	Low (1.4)
3 or more previous births	Low (1.5)	Very low (0.6)	Very low (0.8)	Very low (0.9)	Low (1.5)	Very low (0.9)	Low (1.2)
Under 30 years with 1 or 2 previous births	Moderate (2.0)	Low (1.3)	Very low (0.0)	Low (1.9)	Low (1.7)	Low (1.5)	Low (1.8)
30 and over with 1 or 2 previous births	Very low (0.7)	Very low (0.1)	Very low (0.0)	Low (1.0)	Very low (0.7)	Very low (0.6)	Low (1.1)

Numbers in brackets give the risk for every 100 IUD users during the first year of use
* For definition of 'high', 'moderate' and 'low', see page 00
** Insufficient fittings

be much higher if the IUD is removed and other contraceptive cover not obtained.

It is important that if you miss a period, or otherwise suspect you are pregnant, you should consult your doctor as soon as possible. In many cases the suspicion of pregnancy is not supported and in the small number of cases where a pregnancy is confirmed, the earlier this is known the better. The choices to be made in such a situation become increasingly restricted as the weeks go by, and to delay may be dangerous.

Outcome of an unintended pregnancy

Among the small number of IUD users who do inadvertently become pregnant, the choice of whether to continue with the pregnancy or to seek a termination of the pregnancy is not an easy one to make. Doubtless, the doctor who confirms the pregnancy will discuss the alternative courses of action available. Studies of the experience of IUD users who inadvertently become pregnant have shown that a majority opt for an early termination of the pregnancy, but there is also a sizeable number who decide against this. For those who wish to continue with the pregnancy it is advisable to confirm whether or not the IUD is still in place. If the IUD threads are not visible in the vagina this does not necessarily mean that the IUD is no longer in the uterus. As the uterus enlarges with the pregnancy, the threads can be gradually drawn up into the cervical canal until they disappear from the vagina. In this case a physical examination will not be sufficient to show whether or not the IUD is still in place, but a technique called 'ultrasound' can be used to locate the IUD and also to demonstrate the exact stage of development of the pregnancy.

In about one-third of all reported cases of pregnancy, the IUD is not present. This indicates that the IUD had already been expelled but that the woman had not noticed. In the other two-thirds of the cases where the IUD is still present in the uterus, a decision has to be made about whether to leave it there or to remove it. If the IUD is left in the uterus there is only a 50/50 chance that the pregnancy will end in a full-term birth. The likelihood of miscarriage is much higher in IUD pregnancies than in 'normal' pregnancies. This is because the IUD may interfere with the growth and development of the placenta (or afterbirth) and of the membranes which surround the growing foetus. Most miscarriages occur during the first three months, or first 'trimester' of pregnancy, but some also occur later on. Miscarriages which take place during the second trimester (months 4-6) are usually more serious and more liable to complications than those which take place earlier. Among IUD users the experience of a second trimester miscarriage is about twenty-five times higher than that experienced by pregnant women who had not used an IUD.

If the IUD is removed early in the pregnancy this high rate of miscarriage can be considerably reduced. Studies have shown that if the IUD is removed during the first three months of pregnancy, the miscarriage rate can be cut by one-half, and the incidence of second trimester miscarriages can be almost totally eliminated. For this reason the doctor will usually advise removal of the device, provided the threads are visible and there is no undue difficulty in the removal. If resistance is felt when gently pulling the threads, or if the threads are not visible, the doctor will usually advise that the IUD should be left in place as any attempt at removal would be more likely to induce a miscarriage.

For the pregnancies which proceed for the full nine months, neither the birth process nor the baby itself is at any increased risk because of the presence of the IUD. The whereabouts of the IUD should be ascertained at the time of delivery. It will normally come away with the afterbirth, but there are occasional reports of the device remaining in the uterus. About a third of devices are not found at the time of delivery; this suggests that they were expelled without being noticed before the pregnancy started. It is important that a woman's obstetrician should know during the pregnancy that an IUD is being worn so that appropriate antenatal care can be given. There is no danger of the IUD harming the baby itself or causing any malformations or deformities. This is because the IUD will be outside the sac of amniotic fluid which surrounds and protects the growing baby. Old wives' tales about a baby being born clutching an IUD in its hand, or having the shape of the IUD imprinted on its head are just that – old wives' tales! However, as in any pregnancy, there is always a small risk that the baby will be born handicapped in some way. Very rarely a disturbing enquiry is received from a mother who has tragically given birth to a disabled child, and who feels that the IUD was somehow the cause of the disability. What evidence there is suggests that the risk of giving birth to a malformed child is less for a pregnant IUD wearer than for a woman who is not wearing an IUD. The reasons why this should be so are not certain, but it seems likely that for a baby to survive through the very early stages of its development and implantation in the uterus, it must be particularly robust to be able to deal with the presence of the IUD. If the baby survives the pregnancy in the presence of an IUD and a full-term birth takes place, the odds of the child being malformed are very remote and certainly less than that found in the general population.

Ectopic pregnancy

There is another complication of pregnancy which is of particular importance to the IUD user; this is the increased incidence of ectopic pregnancy among women who become pregnant while wearing an IUD. An ectopic pregnancy is one which takes place *outside* the uterus. The most common site for an ectopic pregnancy to occur is in one of the fallopian tubes. As the embryo grows, the tube will become distended and, if the embryo is allowed to continue to grow, the tube will eventually rupture. This causes severe pain and bleeding and is a serious and life-threatening emergency.

Reliable information about the incidence of ectopic pregnancy is hard to find because of the small numbers involved, and because of uncertainty about the effect of a variety of factors which are difficult to separate out. These factors include the mother's age; number of previous pregnancies; previous miscarriages; social group; racial origin; history of pelvic infection; history of ectopic pregnancy, and various abnormalities of the uterus or the fallopian tubes. One review has shown that there is about a tenfold range in the incidence of ectopic pregnancy among women not wearing an IUD depending on these factors. Previous pelvic infection is thought to be a particularly important factor.

As a general rule, about 1 ectopic pregnancy occurs in every 250 pregnancies. However, this rate is greatly increased to about

1 in every 25 pregnancies among women who become pregnant whilst wearing an IUD. If there is an increased risk of infection among some women wearing an IUD (see the comments on infection) and if infection is believed to be a significant factor in ectopic pregnancy, then a link between IUD use and ectopic pregnancy appears to be logical. But infection is not the whole story and the link between IUD use and a raised incidence of ectopic pregnancy has been observed for at least twenty years. The ratio of 1:25 is an average only and there is some evidence to suggest that this figure varies depending on the type of IUD being worn as well as with the general incidence of pelvic infection in the community. When comparing the IUD with other methods of family planning it is noticeable that an increased risk of an ectopic pregnancy also occurs among women who take the progestogen-only pill (the mini-pill) and those who have been sterilised by tubal ligation.

When considering the risk of ectopic pregnancy it must be remembered that the unwanted pregnancy rates among IUD users are already very low. The 1 in 25 ectopic to uterine pregnancies that occur in this group means that less than 1 in every 1,000 IUD users is likely to experience this complication. Nevertheless, a ruptured ectopic pregnancy is a serious emergency and it is important for a woman wearing an IUD to seek medical advice right away if she misses a period or otherwise suspects she may be pregnant. Doctors are well aware of the increased risk of ectopic pregnancy and will take account of this when making a diagnosis. The usual signs of an early ectopic pregnancy are: delayed menstruation, low abdominal pain and tenderness, and abnormal vaginal bleeding. These symptoms do not necessarily mean an ectopic pregnancy has occurred, but if they do arise an urgent medical check is necessary. If the usual clinic doctor is not available for any reason, the woman should contact another doctor or the emergency department of a local hospital. An ectopic pregnancy is serious and any delay is dangerous.

Perforation of the uterus

A perforation of the uterus occurs when the IUD is inadvertently pushed into and sometimes through the muscular wall of the uterus. It is a very rare event affecting about 1 in every 1,000 and in almost every case occurs at the time of the IUD fitting. Several factors may combine to allow this to happen, including the condition and size of the uterus, the type of device being fitted and the experience of the doctor fitting the IUD. If the uterine muscle is in a relaxed and 'soft' state (perhaps after pregnancy), then extra care needs to be taken at the time of IUD fitting. The IUD itself may have a pointed end which can penetrate the wall of the uterus – again great care has to be taken in fitting such an IUD. With experience over a number of years, most IUD manufacturers now recognise this danger and ensure that the risk of perforation is reduced by careful design of new IUD models. The skill of the doctor fitting the IUD is much harder to measure, but as most uterine perforations occur at the time the IUD is fitted it is this skill which researchers believe to be the most important factor. The woman is usually unaware that a perforation has taken place and this extremely rare occurrence only comes to light when a check-up visit reveals that the IUD is missing. In these rare instances the removal of the IUD usually involves surgery.

Death

Instances of death associated with IUD are extremely rare; only four cases have ever been reported in the UK. In nearly twenty years of research, while collecting one of the largest sets of information about IUDs in the world, involving the experiences of tens of thousands of IUD users, there have been no notifications of IUD-related deaths among women being followed up by the UK IUD Research Network.

Conclusion

This chapter has not been an easy one to write or, presumably, to read as it has dwelt on all the things which can possibly go wrong when a woman is wearing an IUD. It would of course be dishonest and unethical to gloss over these problems; but a chapter such as this tends to stress the problems and so can give a distorted picture of IUD use. As a result, it is easy to gain the impression that the IUD is more dangerous and unpleasant to use than it really is. Having described the pitfalls, it cannot be emphasised too strongly that these problems are only experienced by a minority of women. And these problems must be viewed in the light of the problems which can be caused by using other methods of contraception. The side effects of IUD use tend to be localised to the reproductive system; many women, particularly older women, find these local side effects more acceptable than the risk of the more generalised side effects which are associated with oral contraception.

For the majority of women who have had a baby and who have an IUD fitted, the IUD provides a satisfactory method of contraception and has many advantages: it is a relatively permanent method of contraception, and once fitted it can be forgotten about apart from a routine annual check-up; it is an efficient means of contraception and the likelihood of getting pregnant is quite small; it does not interrupt the sex act or interfere with love-making and so, with fear of pregnancy removed, relationships may be enhanced and enriched.

CHAPTER 6

The history of the IUD

It has been claimed that the use of the IUD can be traced right back to the ancient Greeks when Hippocrates and Soranos recommended the insertion into the vagina of small balls, made of various substances, to support a prolapsed uterus. Hippocrates in his book 'Diseases of Women' mentions a hollow lead tube which could be used to place medicines in the uterus. The tube was presumably used to ensure that such medicines were safely delivered through the vagina and cervical canal. This is often quoted as an illustration of the antiquity of placing substances in the uterus, although there is no evidence that Hippocrates intended any contraceptive action to take place. Much more recently Casanova, whose reputation as a lover was matched by his enthusiasm for testing contraceptive products, also mentions the use of a gold ball which could be placed in the vagina in order to prevent a pregnancy.

Objects like these can hardly be called intrauterine devices; at most, such devices are intravaginal. But the placing of small round stones in the uterus of camels, if true, was definitely an attempt at intrauterine contraception. This alleged forerunner of the IUD of today is almost always mentioned in textbooks and by lecturers giving talks on the history of IUDs. The story goes that nomads about to embark on long caravan journeys with their camels across the Gobi desert (other deserts are also mentioned depending on the story-teller) wanted to make certain that there would be no delay in their journey caused by camels becoming pregnant. Of course the long time these journeys took meant that it was not always possible to keep male and female camels apart. At the same time, these camel drivers wanted to protect the fertility of their expensive animals so that they would produce offspring in the future at the appropriate time and place. And so small round stones (which could be removed at the end of the journey) were placed in the uterus of the female camels. What gave these caravan masters the idea of placing stones in the camel's uterus in the first place is never suggested! Attempts to discover the original source of this often repeated story have not been successful; this led one author to claim that 'the evidence, like the camels themselves, vanishes into the vast and uncharted sands of Araby'. It's a good story though.

Another historical source relates the modern IUD to the use of intracervical and intrauterine stems and pessaries in the last century. These appliances varied in design but usually consisted of some form of ring which remained in the vagina, and a stem which protruded into the cervical canal, or sometimes the uterine cavity itself. These devices were meant to correct flexions and distortions in the position of the uterus which were thought to give rise to complaints such as painful periods or infertility. It is probably true that some physicians fitting these stems and pessaries did so with the aim of preventing pregnancy rather than dealing with gynaecological disorders as was usually claimed. It is worth remembering that the medical profession was opposed to any form of birth control at that time and it was not until well into the present century that there was an official change of mind. In 1878 a Dr Routh roundly condemned the reported use of stem pessaries as contraceptive devices. Speaking to his colleagues at a Bristol Medical Association meeting he did not mince his words. He claimed that the use of the intrauterine stem 'implies the assistance of a person of some skill, and shows to what degree of degradation some men have fallen. The question presents itself – "Who put them there?"'. One can imagine him glaring over his spectacles as his eyes swept over his audience of professional colleagues.

The publicity which followed such an outburst probably increased the use of such devices for contraceptive purposes. Nevertheless, the professional discussions about family planning and birth control at that time remained hostile. Perhaps Dr Routh would not be pleased to see the changes that have occurred in the hundred years since his condemnation in 1878 – but Dr Albutt would be pleased. Dr Arthur Albutt was struck off the medical register in 1887 because he assisted in the publication of a booklet which contained a section on 'How to prevent conception when advised by the Doctor'. It is ironic that less than 100 years ago doctors were putting their professional careers at risk if they were associated with the fitting of an IUD, whereas today doctors have a virtual monopoly on IUD fittings.

One difficulty in tracing the historical developments of IUDs in this way is that the stem pessary was the name given to a wide range of devices intended for a variety of uses. In addition to providing support for a prolapsed womb, they were also used to encourage fertility by holding open the cervix, or by holding the uterus upright. As we have seen, some did not enter the uterus or cervix at all and merely rested in the vagina. Whilst not denying that some stem pessaries could have been used with contraception in mind, they were not really IUDs.

To find the first published report of a device that could legitimately be called an IUD, we have to go back to September 1909 when a short two-page report appeared in a German medical journal, written by a doctor called Richard Richter. In this report he described his use of a flexible silkworm-gut ring, made up of two twisted strands and about 25 mm (1 inch) in diameter. He had placed this flexible ring into the uterus of women seeking contraceptive advice at his medical practice in Waldenburg, just outside Breslau. Richter did not give details of how many women he had fitted with this device or of how successful it was in preventing pregnancies. However, he must have been fitting IUDs for some years because he also described his lack of success using a single coil of silkworm gut before adopting the double coil version he was now reporting. Richter was enthusiastic about this 'new' method of contraception and was willing to discuss it openly, even though there was general condemnation of contraception at that time. But nothing more was heard from Dr Richter and the subject of IUDs was almost totally ignored for a further twenty years.

There now arrived on to the stage another famous name in the history of IUDs. In 1929 Dr Ernst Grafenberg reported his work using an 18 mm gut ring, later adapted and made of silver wire. He claimed that the only way to prevent the infection which had always been associated with the use of stem pessaries, was to place a device wholly within the uterus. He indicated that this idea was not new, but he did not refer to Richter by name. This new report about intrauterine contraception coincided with the growth of the birth control movement and the establishment of birth control clinics, whose aim was to improve the health and living conditions of women generally. It was for this reason that Grafenberg's ideas reached a wide audience. The public debate was intense and acrimonious. There were two main reasons why the controversy concerning IUDs continued even when the birth control movement was visibly gathering strength. The IUD was not differentiated from the stem pessary in the minds of most people. There was ignorance of how the IUD worked (an ignorance not entirely overcome today) and a general dislike even by most doctors of openly discussing sexual matters. In addition, the problem of infection and of pelvic inflammatory disease during this pre-antibiotic era was serious, and it was stressed time and again in the medical literature of the time. It was unfortunate that at the time Grafenberg presented his paper, the incidence of pelvic inflammatory disease was on the increase in Europe. The Grafenberg Ring, despite yielding a very low pregnancy rate of 1.6 for every 100 women using the device, gradually fell into disrepute and by 1935 was largely discredited.

For the next two decades little was heard of the IUD; between 1935 and 1959 only one publication appeared in the English language which was about IUDs. But during this period the fitting of IUDs was continuing quietly. Jackson in England was using the Grafenberg Ring, and Hall in the USA was fitting a stainless steel ring, but neither of these gynaecologists made their work known until the 1960s. Ota, in Japan, had been using a modified Grafenberg Ring since 1934 and this device, known by his name, is still in use in Japan today.

The work of Dr Margaret Jackson is of particular interest for it subsequently led to the first major evaluation of IUDs in the United Kingdom. The circumstances surrounding Dr Jackson's first fitting of a Grafenberg Ring illustrates the difficulties facing doctors during the early years of contraceptive provision. In the 1930s the only methods of family planning generally available were the cap or diaphragm and the sheath. Spermicides were available but they were not regarded as very effective. Abortion was illegal and the resulting poor health of women because of too many pregnancies, or the effects of 'back-street' abortions was a serious problem. The arrival of the IUD has to be seen against such a background to appreciate its significance. Dr Jackson's experience demonstrates the difficulties facing a conscientious and socially minded doctor at that time.

A farmer, who was the father of a mentally handicapped girl, sought Dr Jackson's advice about the behaviour of his young, unmarried daughter who had developed a healthy sexual appetite. Two babies had already been born and he was keen to avoid a third. The alternatives were to keep the girl locked up at home, or to send her away. The father loved his daughter and saw no reason for locking her away; what was to be done? Dr Jackson had heard, and read, about the intrauterine device invented by Dr Ernst Grafenberg and after some thought and consultation she fitted her first Grafenberg Ring. Much has happened since that fitting in a Devon farmhouse. Dr Jackson is now retired, but she has gained an international reputation with her work on IUDs. The farmer's daughter could have had no idea of the national and international repercussions of her adventures, now so long ago.

The silence about IUD use was broken in 1959 when the editors of the *American Journal of Obstetrics and Gynaecology* published a paper by an Israeli gynaecologist – Oppenheimer – describing twenty years of experience of fitting various types of IUD. By coincidence, in the same year, an article was published in a Japanese medical journal describing the use of the Ota Ring by over 20,000 women in Japan. Both these papers reported low pregnancy rates and an absence of serious side effects. This work by Oppenheimer and Ishihama interested the Population Council, an American organisation which had been set up in 1954 to study various aspects of population growth and which was looking for a safe and efficient method of birth control for use in developing countries. As a result, the first international conference on IUDs took place in New York during April 1962.

This meeting attracted just forty-eight interested workers who got together to discuss experiences with various IUDs and to determine the direction of future IUD research. Participants, including Dr Jackson, gave details of their clinical experience and all indicated that serious side effects were few; there was no evidence of cancer related to IUD use, and there was no impairment of fertility after IUD removal. Some disadvantages were mentioned but, on balance, the advantages far outweighed any discernible disadvantages. Here was a method of family planning which could be used for large numbers of women in national family planning programmes.

A number of different types of device were discussed at the 1962 meeting. Some silk-gut coils were made by hand, and similar to those developed by Richter and Grafenberg; others were made of stainless steel or silver wire. But the most interesting were the devices made of plastic with their shapes moulded in the form of spirals, coils or loops. The use of a plastic material allowed the introduction of devices which could be straightened out and loaded into a small bore introducer. The small size introducer, unlike the much larger devices which previously had to be inserted through the cervix, caused much less pain and discomfort at the time of fitting. The advantages for both patient and doctor were immediately obvious.

These plastic devices also had a 'memory' in that once the device was pushed out of the introducer into the uterine cavity, the device took up its original shape once again. This development was very important, and since that time almost all devices have been designed in this way. The first device of this type was the Margulie's Spiral, but the idea was soon adapted in the production of the more common 'Lippes Loop'.

The Lippes Loop also had a nylon thread attached to one end of the device. This thread allowed for easier removal of the device whenever this was desired. The presence of the thread also gave assurance that the device was in the correct place and presumably doing its job of preventing unwanted pregnancies. Since the early 1960s, the Lippes Loop has probably become the most widely distributed IUD in the world. Most people simply know the IUD as the 'loop', after the device Jack Lippes publicised in 1962.

There is another reason why this 1962 New York conference was important. There was a need for a scientific study, designed to evaluate the clinical information being gathered about IUDs. Investigators were using different techniques, different definitions of likely side effects, and even different statistical procedures when they reported their experience. What was needed was a study that could coordinate this information in such a way that reliance could be placed on the accuracy of the reports being made. It was largely as a result of the 1962 conference that Christopher Tietze instituted his now famous study called 'The Cooperative Statistical Program for the Evaluation of Contraceptive Devices'. This title was inevitably shortened and became known simply as the 'CSP'. The CSP started in 1963 and continued until 1968 when the collection of information ceased, although reports continued to be published for some years afterwards. The object of the CSP was to provide detailed statistical analysis of IUD use and effectiveness, and it was unique in that uniform procedures and a systematic statistical approach in evaluation were used for the first time. The contributors to the CSP were obliged to conform to rigorous standards of information collection and reporting. Most of the collaborators were in the USA, but there were just three from other parts of the world – Sweden, Fiji and England. The English data was supplied by the Exeter Family Planning Clinic whose senior medical officer was the indefatigable worker, Dr Margaret Jackson. Almost 32,000 women were included in the CSP, providing over half-a-million 'woman-months' of observation. It was a gigantic study and it has been the basis of information about IUDs ever since.

During the early period of the CSP a second international meeting was called (in 1964) and this led the way to the international distribution and use of IUDs which has continued ever since. It should be remembered that the IUD was being actively promoted at the same time as fears about the growing size of the world population were being expressed. In the 1950s and 1960s attempts were being made to introduce family planning programmes which would slow down the rapid rate of the world population increase. At that time it was argued that the availability of food and other resources in the world would not keep pace with the continually increasing number of people who required to be fed, clothed, housed and supplied with energy. A major hurdle in the introduction of these family planning programmes was the lack of an effective and easily provided contraceptive method. The oral contraceptive had just been invented but this new method required daily motivation to take it properly. The diaphragm or cap was often disliked and sometimes ineffective. The sheath was not popular because it required cooperation from the male partner and also because it had an association with promiscuity. The IUD appeared to population planners as an answer to all their problems. It was effective and relatively safe; it did not require daily motivation in its use, nor education in how to use it properly and, once in place, it would continue to exert its contraceptive effect from year to year. We now know that the IUD was not the hoped-for resolution of all family planning problems, but it does have one characteristic which has probably done more to encourage its use in family planning programmes than anything else. Put simply, if the IUD is fitted in January and it is seen to be in place the following July then the observer knows it should have been doing its job during February, March, April, May and June. Those responsible for assessing the effectiveness of contraceptives had come across a method which, when an unintended pregnancy occurred, would enable them to answer the basic question 'Is it the method of contraception that is at fault, or is it the poor use of the method by the person using it?' The pill, the cap or diaphragm and the sheath always left these questions partly unanswered because the person assessing the effectiveness of the method could never be sure that the method was being used correctly. In IUD use, the 'human' factors associated with ineffective use no longer applied.

This digression from the history of the IUD is not made merely to make an interesting point; the ability to collect accurate statistical information about the method, and the ability to remove the vagaries of human behaviour or memory from the equation, led to the international use of the IUD in a big way. Some authors in the 1960s claimed that the IUD was the answer to the world population problem. All that was needed was the mass fitting of IUDs in countries where overpopulation was present and the IUD could be left – quietly and inexpensively – to do its work.

But this view, both of the population problem and of the IUD as a means of solving it, is over-simplistic; it was not long before the shortcomings of the concept of population control and of the

IUD were recognised. The view that the IUD would be an acceptable method of family planning for everybody had to be modified when it was realised that many women objected to the IUD fitting. Apart from the inconvenience of the IUD fitting itself, the introduction of administrative procedures designed to recruit sufficient numbers of women from a 'target' population rapidly gave the impression of an official drive for population control irrespective of the feelings of those for whom the IUD service was intended. 'Educational' campaigns and inducements of various kinds served only to reinforce this impression of official compulsion. For any family planning method to be used effectively over a sustained period of time, a personal commitment is necessary, and this requires a positive realisation that the use of such a family planning method will increase the quality of life of the individual concerned. While reducing the need for daily motivation, the IUD still required the cooperation of the user to have it fitted in the first place, and to put up with side effects not normally experienced. Any suggestion of population control or of a denial of personal choice was counter productive, and the presence of medical teams and the experience of a minor operative procedure reinforced this suggestion.

A second problem was that the IUD, while being effective in preventing unwanted pregnancies, had the side effect of increasing blood loss at the time of menstruation. The dislike of this side effect led many women to demand the removal of the IUD following earlier agreement to its fitting. The effect of disturbed menstrual bleeding on the social, religious and personal life of many women was profound. After early enthusiasm for the IUD in family planning programmes in many parts of the world, the method did not live up to the optimistic claims being made for it.

The next major breakthrough occurred in the late 1960s when copper was added to the plastic devices. It was found that with the addition of fine copper wire wound around the plastic stem of the device, the device could be made to a smaller size without increasing the risk of pregnancy. The first examples were in the form of a number 7 and the letter T; the Copper 7 and the Copper T have been known by these names ever since. The inventors were a Chilean doctor, Jaime Zipper, and an American medical researcher, Howard Tatum. Both had been experimenting with the use of different metals for a number of years. Dr Zipper noticed that when he placed a small amount of copper wire in the uterus of a rabbit, the rabbit did not become pregnant despite an active sex life. He concluded that the copper wire was reacting with the lining of the uterus making it inhospitable to the passage of sperm or a fertilised ovum. The copper-carrying device invented by Dr Zipper had one major advantage: the device could give the same protection against pregnancy but the size of the device could be greatly reduced. The smaller the IUD, then the smaller the IUD inserter; and the smaller the bore of the inserter, the less the discomfort experienced by the woman at IUD fitting. This meant that a woman who had not previously given birth could now be fitted with an IUD, where previously such women had found the fitting experience too uncomfortable.

Copper devices do, however, have one disadvantage: the copper gradually disintegrates and it is necessary to remove a copper device and refit a new one at routine intervals. This interval varies with the type of device and the recommendations of the manufacturer, but is normally every two to five years. The rate at which the copper disintegrates varies from woman to woman, and there is no evidence that protection against pregnancy is reduced as the copper gradually disintegrates. There is, therefore, still some uncertainty about the longest time a copper device can safely be left in place before a routine change becomes really necessary. More recently, solid copper 'sleeves' or 'bands' have been used in the design of the newer devices, instead of using copper wire. The use of this more solid form of copper is intended to reduce the amount of fragmentation occurring, and so prolong the life of the IUD so that less frequent changing of devices is necessary.

During the 1970s, the use of copper-carrying IUDs became commonplace; a new fashion in IUD design had arrived. But it is interesting to see that the unwanted pregnancy rates associated with IUD use were still at about the same level as Grafenberg had been reporting in the 1930s. Nevertheless, the smaller sized IUD was easier to fit, and less uncomfortable to have fitted, and because of this many more women became potential users of the

IUD. At the same time as the number of potential IUD users increased, IUDs also became much more expensive. This was partly because devices were now marketed already pre-sterilised, together with a disposable introducer. It is hardly surprising that the IUD became a serious proposition for investment and development.

In the United Kingdom, it was as copper-carrying IUDs were becoming popular in the early 1970s that changes occurred in the organisation and administration of family planning clinics. Since the 1930s, the Family Planning Association had been setting up and running family planning clinics on a voluntary and charitable basis. Throughout this time there had been a sustained campaign to lobby for free family planning services provided within the National Health Service. In 1974 the goal of free family planning provision was at last achieved, and almost all family planning clinics were taken over by local health authorities. In the following year arrangements were also made for the family doctor to provide family planning services. This meant that the fitting of IUDs was no longer confined to a specially trained group of clinic doctors. No agreement was reached concerning the level or duration of training required, and ten years on there is still no requirement that doctors fitting IUDs should be required to undergo initial or periodic training. Most doctors who fit IUDs do undertake such training voluntarily, and the organisations concerned about doctors' training and the provision of family planning services continue to press for a proper registration of doctors who wish to provide an IUD service. As a result of cuts in the funding of local health services, some authorities have considered closing down family planning clinics as an economy measure. They argue that as family doctors are now able to provide family planning services, the clinics just duplicate this provision and are therefore unnecessary. However, research has shown that this is not the case; whilst almost all GPs provide the pill, relatively few fit IUDs – and those who do, fit relatively few devices. Family planning clinics are still important for the provision of IUDs, and as a specialist referral centre for women who experience problems with other methods of contraception.

After the copper-carrying IUDs have come the hormone-releasing IUDs. These more modern devices not only prevent pregnancy, but also release hormones that reduce the incidence of unwanted bleeding and of expulsion. The device contains a semi-permeable membrane which permits the slow release of the hormone carried within it at a precise and pre-determined rate. The hormone-releasing IUDs are really of the next century and indicate the direction in which the provision of medicine may go in the future.

This then is the history of the IUD. The story is not complete for progress is still being made in the search for the IUD that is easy and painless to fit, does not expel, is comfortable to use, is easy and painless to remove, does not lead to undesirable side effects and above all, provides confidence to the user that an unwanted pregnancy will not occur.

CHAPTER 7
Research findings

The research findings discussed here are confined to the experience of IUD users wearing devices in common use in Europe or America at the present time. The information about the risks of unplanned pregnancy, rejection of the IUD leading to expulsion from the uterus, and removal of the IUD following complaints of bleeding and/or pain has been collected by the UK IUD Research Network. This organisation consists of twenty-three senior family planning doctors who have together been responsible for the care of many thousands of IUD users in the last ten years. This information relates to the 'ordinary' IUD users attending family planning clinics situated in a variety of towns and cities throughout England, Scotland and Wales. The fitting of the IUD and subsequent experience of these women will have been typical of that expected for any group of IUD users.

The information given in the following pages is about specific IUD models, but first it is vital to consider the most important general issues which have arisen from the research findings of the last fifteen years. These may be summarised as follows:

1) The IUD has a high level of effectiveness in preventing pregnancy. On average there are between 1 and 2 pregnancies among every 100 IUD users during the first year of use, with a gradual decline in this risk of unplanned pregnancy the longer the IUD is worn.
2) Expulsion of the device from the uterus will occur in less than 10 per cent of IUD users; the precise risk depends on the type of IUD and the age and parity of the user. There is a dramatic fall in the rate of expulsion within a month or two of fitting, and very few expulsions take place after the first six months of use.

3) The removal of the IUD following complaints of pain or of a disturbed menstrual cycle occurs in about 10 per cent of IUD users, depending on the device being worn and the age and parity of the user. There is a slow but steady decrease in this type of complaint the longer the IUD is worn.

4) IUDs are safe provided prompt advice is sought if any unusual side effects are experienced. This is particularly important if a menstrual period is missed or if lower abdominal pain or tenderness is experienced. Heavy or prolonged menstrual bleeding and any abnormal vaginal discharge should also be reported promptly.

5) Women who have already given birth to a child appear to be more suited to IUD use than women who have not yet borne a child.

6) Women who have a history of pelvic infection, previous ectopic pregnancy, heavy menstrual bleeding, rheumatic heart disease, or who are currently taking drugs for any condition should make sure that the doctor knows about this when making a decision about IUD use.

7) The small number of IUD users who become pregnant while wearing an IUD are more likely to experience an ectopic pregnancy than other women.

8) The side effects most commonly associated with IUD use are increased menstrual bleeding and discomfort.

9) IUD use is associated with a higher risk of pelvic infection. This may be due to the inability of the IUD to prevent infection taking place. IUD users are at increased risk if they have more than one sexual partner. Pelvic infection can lead to subsequent infertility and should be treated promptly.

10) Who fits the IUD is as important a factor as which IUD is fitted, in terms of the risk of unplanned pregnancy or other unwanted side effects.

11) Satisfaction with the IUD as a means of contraception depends to a great extent on the age and parity of the IUD user.

12) In general, the risk of an unplanned pregnancy does not appear to have been significantly lowered since the 1960s, despite changes in IUD design.
13) Expulsion of the IUD from the uterus has been significantly reduced with newer IUD designs.
14) Copper-carrying IUDs tend to be smaller in size and are therefore less uncomfortable to fit. The pregnancy rate is similar to that of other IUDs; but they appear to cause a smaller increase of menstrual bleeding.
15) The major issues involved in IUD fitting and use include: degrees of discomfort at fitting; ability to prevent unplanned pregnancy; likelihood of expulsion from the uterus; likelihood of removal because of an unwanted side effect; and ease of removal when this is desired. All these should be considered when evaluating a specific IUD model.
16) No single IUD model in general use appears to be significantly better or worse than other models when all of these major issues are considered together.

DEFINITIONS OF RISK

The definitions given below are used in the following pages to describe the risk of pregnancy, expulsion, or device removal during the first year of IUD use among every 100 IUD users.

PREGNANCY
Very low: less than 1
Low: between 1 and 2
Moderate: between 2 and 4
High: 5 or more

EXPULSION
Very low: less than 3
Low: between 3 and 4
Moderate: between 5 and 9
High: 10 or more

REMOVAL
Very low: less than 3
Low: between 3 and 4
Moderate: between 5 and 9
High: 10 or more

The Gravigard (Copper 7) IUD

Description

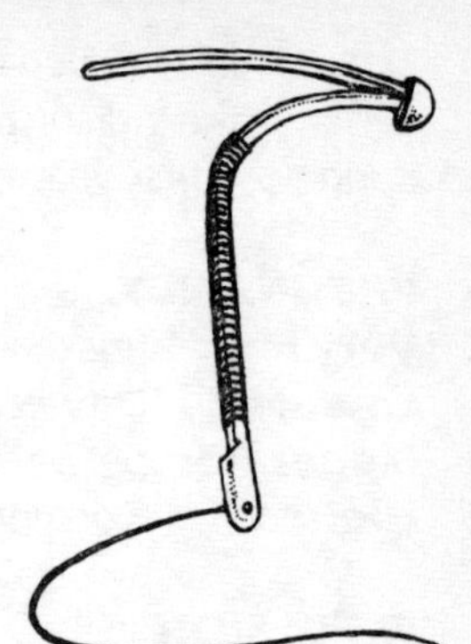

The Gravigard (or Copper 7) is designed in the shape of a figure 7 and has 200 square mm of fine copper wire wound round the vertical stem. The device is made of plastic with barium sulphate added to make it more easily seen on X-ray should this be required.

The device is 36 mm long and 26 mm wide.

The device is loaded into the inserter tube by placing the stem and folding the arm of the '7' into the top of the tube. The half-round join where the stem and arm meet rests on the top of the inserter tube giving a total diameter of slightly over 3 mm as the device and inserter pass through the cervical canal. The Gravigard is either pushed into the uterus by an inner rod inside the inserter tube, or held steady by the internal rod while the inserter tube is withdrawn over it. (See Chapter 4 for more detail.)

The recommended period of use is two years (UK) or three years (USA).

The Mini-Gravigard is identical to the standard Gravigard but with the stem and arm being only four-fifths the standard size.

Table 4 Experience during the first year of 15,097 women fitted with the Gravigard (Copper 7) IUD in one of the UK IUD Research Network Clinics

Type of IUD user	Pregnancy risk	Expulsion risk	Removal for bleeding/pain
No previous birth	Low (1.2)	High (11.1)	Moderate (7.9)
1 or 2 previous births	Low (1.7)	High (10.0)	Moderate (8.9)
3 or more previous births	Low (1.5)	Moderate (6.0)	Moderate (8.3)

Numbers in brackets give the level of risk among every 100 women wearing the Gravigard (Copper 7) IUD using Life Table Analysis techniques

Comment

This IUD was first introduced in 1974 from the USA using a design developed in Chile. It was designed to fold into the smallest size inserter tube possible and so cause the minimum amount of discomfort at the time of fitting. This was achieved and reports of pain at the time of fitting and removal are rare. But the cost of this ease of fitting and removal is the relatively high risk of expulsion experienced by the women wearing this device. The Gravigard is known to be difficult to place exactly at the fundus (or top) of the uterus and this may explain the relatively high expulsion rate. Many of the expulsions are only 'partial'; that is, the device has moved to lie partly in the cervical canal. Often these partial expulsions are discovered only at the time of a follow-up examination. Table 4 demonstrates that there is a decrease in the risk of expulsion among those Gravigard users who have had three or more children. Women who have not had a baby are almost twice as likely to expel this device. The same is true of increasing age: the older the Gravigard user the lower the risk of expulsion. As with other IUDs, the expulsion risk falls very rapidly after a few months and continues to decrease with time. The pregnancy risk also reduces over time and a decrease takes place in the complaints of bleeding and menstrual discomfort, but this decrease is much more gradual.

If the Gravigard is routinely refitted after two or three years of use there is a partial return to the first year level of risks, but these rapidly return to the level which would be expected had the device not been changed.

The small-size Gravigard has been worn by only a few nulliparous women in the UK. Research shows that the expulsion risk is halved during the first year of use compared with the standard size, but unfortunately removal of the device following a complaint of bleeding or pain is doubled.

The Gyne T (Copper T) IUD

Description

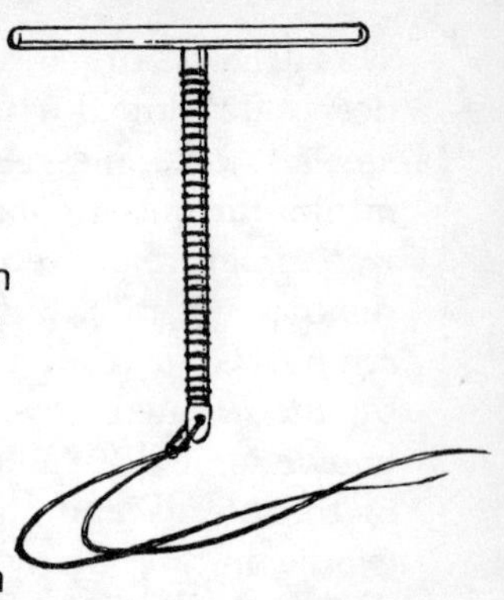

The Copper T has a stem and two arms and as the name suggests is shaped like the letter T. It was developed in 1972 and was the first device to incorporate the addition of copper wire into its design. It was a much smaller sized device than those available at that time and depended on the release of copper ions in the uterus to supplement its contraceptive effect. The device is made of plastic, is 36 mm long and 32 mm wide when in the uterus and 4.4 mm wide when the arms are folded into the inserter tube ready for passing through the cervical canal. The most common version of the Copper T has 200 square mm of fine copper wire wound around the vertical stem. Some variations of this design have the copper in the form of more solid bands around the stem or arms. In other versions the copper wire has a silver core; these adaptations are intended to prevent fragmentation of the copper.

The Copper T is fitted using the 'push-out' or 'withdrawal' techniques (see Chapter 4).

The most common version is recommended to be replaced every three years.

Table 5 Experience during the first year of 4,622 women fitted with the Gyne T (Copper T) IUD in one of the UK IUD Research Network Clinics

Type of IUD user	Pregnancy risk	Expulsion risk	Removal for bleeding/pain
No previous birth	Very low (0.9)	Moderate (9.3)	Moderate (8.4)
1 or 2 previous births	Very low (0.9)	Moderate (5.5)	Moderate (6.5)
3 or more previous births	Very low (0.6)	Low (3.3)	Low (4.9)

Numbers in brackets give the level of risk among every 100 women wearing the Gyne T (Copper T) IUD using Life Table Analysis techniques

Comment

This American device was the first to carry copper and in terms of the risks of unplanned pregnancy, expulsion of the device from the uterus, and removal following complaints of bleeding or menstrual discomfort, it is relatively successful. By reducing the size of the device (when compared with the earlier Lippes Loop or the Saf-T-Coil), the Copper T also led the way in enabling the wearing of IUDs by women who had not previously had a baby. The smaller size causes less discomfort as the device passes through the cervical canal at the time of fitting and removal. But fitting the Copper T sometimes causes difficulties for the doctor; the arms of the T need to be folded into the top of the inserter tube just before fitting and under sterile conditions, and this is not as simple as it sounds. The manufacturer of the device has distributed a gadget which makes the loading of the device easier, but this has not entirely removed the difficulty. The Copper T continues its high protection against pregnancy, and moderate to low likelihood of expulsion or of causing bleeding disturbance throughout its recommended period of use (three years). As with other devices the risk of expulsion falls dramatically after the first few months. It is interesting to notice how this device performs particularly well in the case of women who have had several children.

With this relatively good performance in preventing unwanted side effects, it is not surprising that this device has a high international reputation, although the numbers fitted in the United Kingdom are not high when compared with other devices.

The Multiload IUD

Description

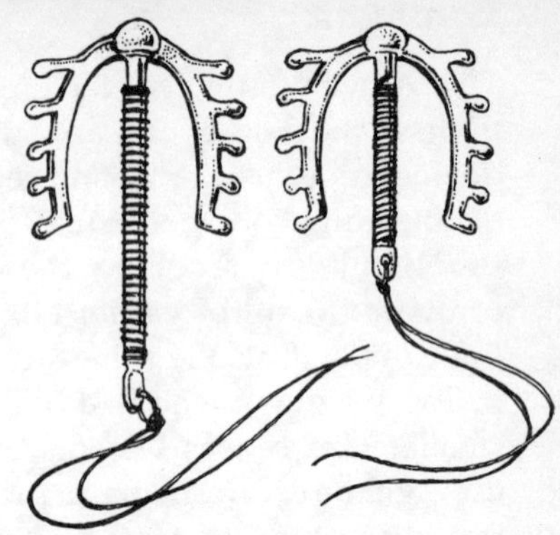

Sometimes called the MLCu250 this device comes in five sizes, but only the 'standard' and 'short' sizes are currently in common use. The 'short' multiload has a shortened vertical stem and a blue (as opposed to a clear) thread, but is otherwise identical to the standard size. Both devices carry 250 square mm of fine copper wire wound around the stem. The arms are flexible and each has five fin-like additions intended to reduce the risk of expulsion of the device from the uterus.

The width of the device is normally between 16 mm and 20.5 mm but this is reduced to 12 mm when the Multiload is passed through the cervical canal.

The device is fitted by placing the vertical stem in the top of a hollow inserter tube; as the device is passed through the cervical canal, its arms fold over the outside of the inserter tube. Once in the uterus, the tube is gently withdrawn leaving the Multiload in place.

The duration of use is at present recommended to be for three years.

Table 6 Experience during the first year of 803 women fitted with the Multiload IUD in one of the UK IUD Research Network Clinics

Type of IUD user	Pregnancy risk	Expulsion risk	Removal for bleeding/pain
No previous birth	Very low (0.0)	Moderate (6.1)	High (10.8)
1 or 2 previous births	Low (1.5)	Moderate (5.4)	Moderate (9.0)
3 or more previous births	Very low (0.9)	Very low (1.7)	High (11.3)

Numbers in brackets give the level of risk among every 100 women wearing the Multiload IUD using Life Table Analysis techniques

Comment

This device was first introduced in 1974 and is one of the few IUDs generally available in the UK which have been developed in Europe; most of the other devices have their origin in the USA. The Multiload was designed to reduce the risk of expulsion from the uterus; the fin-like additions to the arms cause the muscular contractions of the uterus to push the device upwards and farther into the uterus, rather than downwards and out of the uterus through the cervical canal. This design is called 'fundal-seeking' and the figures given in Table 6 would suggest that the design has been relatively successful; the Multiload has one of the lowest risks of expulsion among the IUDs generally available. This is particularly so among women who have had three or more previous pregnancies. The relatively low risk of expulsion is accompanied by a low risk of unplanned pregnancy. This high protection against pregnancy and relatively low likelihood of expulsion continues into the second year and is not only a feature of early use of the device. As the Multiload generally stays in place once it is fitted, it is particularly suitable for women who may find difficulty in attending for follow-up visits.

The Multiload design has not been so successful in eliminating complaints associated with increased bleeding or menstrual discomfort; these complaints are on the high side when compared with other commonly used IUDs. It could be argued that the most important characteristics of an IUD are that it prevents pregnancy and that unnoticed expulsions do not occur. In this the Multiload is successful.

A disadvantage of Multiload use is discomfort at the time of fitting and removal. The width of the device is the largest of any device currently available and this frequently causes a certain amount of discomfort as it passes through the narrow cervical canal. However, this discomfort is transient and most Multiload users experience fitting or removal of the device without undue complaint.

The Novagard IUD

Description

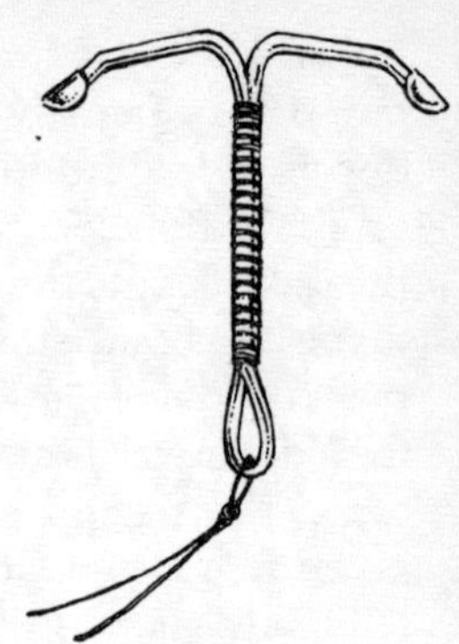

The Novagard (or Nova T) is made of plastic and has 200 square mm of fine copper wire wound around the vertical stem. The wire has a silver core running through its length which is intended to prevent the copper wire fragmenting. This prolongs the period of time during which the Novagard remains effective and obviates the need for frequent routine re-fitting. There is a loop of plastic on the tip of the stem to reduce the risk of expulsion from the uterus. The arms of the device are shaped to form a T when open, but at fitting and removal they bend upwards from the centre and come together to form a single straight line.

The Novagard is 32 mm long and 32 mm wide when open and just 3.6 mm wide when in the inserter tube. The device is fitted using the 'push-out' or 'withdrawal' technique (see Chapter 4).

The recommended period of use is five years.

Table 7 Experience during the first year of 439 women fitted with the Novagard IUD in one of the UK IUD Research Network Clinics

Type of IUD user	Pregnancy risk	Expulsion risk	Removal for bleeding/pain
No previous birth	Moderate (2.2)	Very low (0.0)	Moderate (6.5)
1 or 2 previous births	Very low (0.0)	Low (3.9)	Low (4.4)
3 or more previous births	Very low (0.8)	Low (4.6)	Moderate (6.2)

Numbers in brackets give the level of risk among every 100 women wearing the Novagard IUD. Owing to the relatively small amount of information the Pearl Index has been used to calculate these figures

Comment

Although the Novagard was first developed (in Finland) in 1979, it is the most recent device to be generally available in the UK of all those described. Its design incorporates two important features resulting from the experience of earlier IUDs: it 'closes up' – making it easier to fit and remove, and it carries a type of copper wire which normally gives five years of uninterrupted use. The ability of the device to close up in the way described also suggests that it 'gives' when the muscles of the uterus contract. This means the device copes with normal uterine contractions without being expelled from the uterus. Table 7 shows that the risks of unplanned pregnancy, or expulsion, or disturbed bleeding and menstrual discomfort are favourable when compared with other devices (see Tables 1, 2, and 3 in Chapter 5 where devices are compared).

The Novagard is also easy to load into the sterile inserter tube simply by placing the stem in the top of the tube and pulling on the threads which pass through the tube. The Novagard folds into the inserter automatically without any need to handle the device. The small bore inserter tube (3.6 mm) is conducive to relatively painless fitting. This means that the five major aspects of IUD use (ease of fitting, low risks of pregnancy, expulsion and increased bleeding, and ease of removal) appear to have been achieved. The period of use before a routine re-fitting is required has also been extended with the Novagard. Whereas with other copper-carrying IUDs replacement is advised every two or three years, the Novagard is said to be effective for up to five years of use. More information is required before the UK IUD Research Network can confirm these early promising findings, but present indications are that the Novagard is a very useful device.

The Lippes Loop IUD

Description

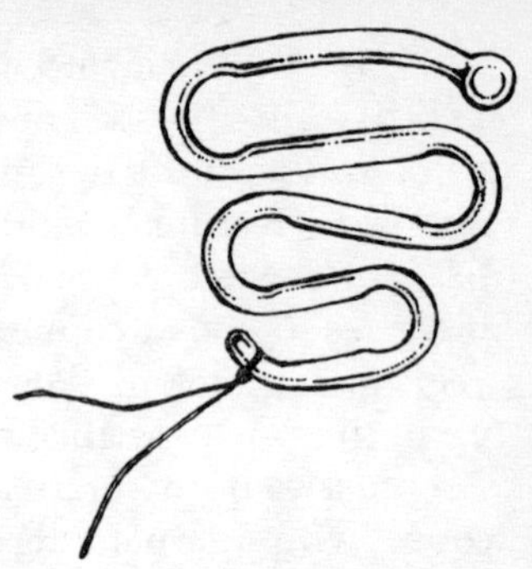

There are four sizes of Lippes Loop, but that shown is size C, the one in most common use. The sizes are labelled A, B, C, D, in increasing size, and with Size D made of a thicker and more rigid material. The devices are made of a plastic-based polymer which is impregnated with a radiopaque material to make them visible on X-ray. The Lippes Loops in general use do not carry copper, but more recently copper bands have been added with the aim of increasing the contraceptive effect.

The length and width of the Lippes Loop C is about 30 mm and the size of the rectangular inserter tube into which it is placed for passing through the cervical canal measures 5 mm by 4 mm. The usual method of placing the device into the uterus is by the 'push' technique (see Chapter 4).

As the device does not normally carry copper wire or bands there is no specific recommendation for the length of time it can be left in the uterus before routine re-fitting is required.

Table 8 Experience during the first year of 8,440 women fitted with the Lippes Loop (C) IUD in one of the UK IUD Research Network Clinics

Type of IUD user	Pregnancy risk	Expulsion risk	Removal for bleeding/pain
No previous birth	**	**	**
1 or 2 previous births	Low (1.0)	Moderate (7.1)	High (10.5)
3 or more previous births	Very low (0.9)	Low (3.6)	Moderate (8.5)

Numbers in brackets give the level of risk among every 100 women wearing the Lippes Loop (C) IUD using Life Table Analysis techniques
** Insufficient fittings

Comment

The Lippes Loop is probably the most well-known device in the history of IUD development. First produced in 1962 by the American doctor whose name it bears, it marked the beginning of the new wave of IUD design that took place during the 1960s. The Lippes Loop design included two important innovative features: first, it could be straightened out and loaded into a narrow inserter tube; second, it had threads attached which allowed its presence to be checked by the user, and which permitted easy removal when this was desired. While not the first IUD to incorporate these advantages, it was the Lippes Loop which became the most widely distributed throughout the world. At the time of its development the wearing of an IUD by women who had not previously given birth to a child was rare because of the discomfort likely to be caused at the time of fitting. Among women who had previously borne children it was a useful contraceptive and many millions were fitted in a variety of family planning programmes. It is still available today, but fitted much less frequently. The device was, and is, successful in preventing pregnancy and carries a moderate risk of expulsion and removal of the device following a complaint of disturbed menstrual bleeding or pain.

The size of Lippes Loop described in table 8 is not usually worn by women who have not already had a baby, and even the smaller sizes (A and B) are not now recommended for such use. However, the women for whom the Lippes Loop was originally intended (those who have borne children) are well protected and research shows that this protection continues in subsequent years. The continuing advantage of the Lippes Loop is that, once fitted, it can be worn indefinitely. For many Lippes Loop users the experience of IUD fitting is a 'once-only' event.

Other IUD models

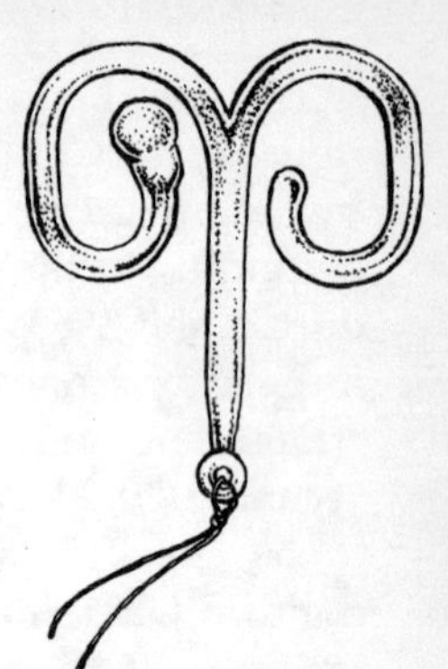

Saf-T-Coil (USA)
This device is no longer manufactured, but many women may still be wearing this device. It has a low pregnancy risk, a moderate risk of expulsion, but a high risk of bleeding disturbance or menstrual discomfort. It does not carry copper and can be worn indefinitely.

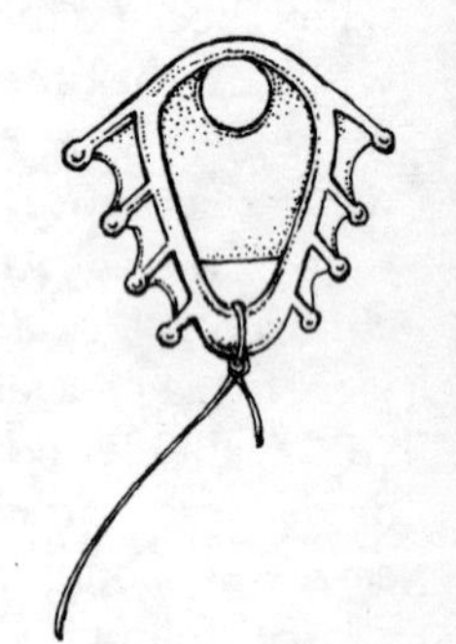

Dalkon Shield (USA)
This device has not been fitted for over ten years and has been withdrawn from use. There has been a great deal of publicity about allegations that its use is directly associated with a very high risk of pelvic infection. Controversy continues about these allegations, with conflicting research evidence being reported.

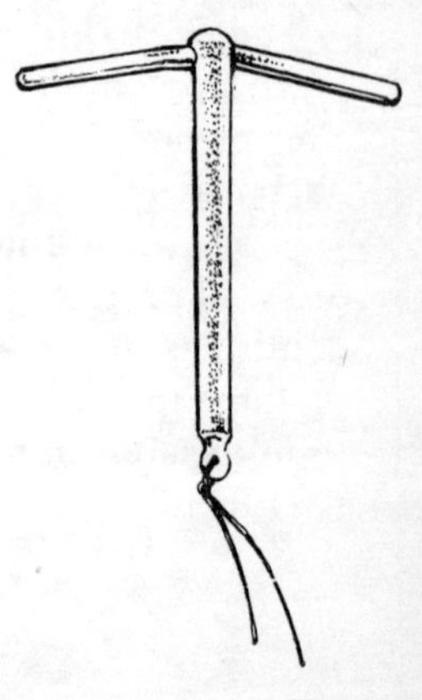

Progestasert (USA)
This IUD is designed to deliver a hormone (progesterone) into the uterus at a fixed rate each day. Its recommended life is twelve to eighteen months and it is considered particularly appropriate for women who normally experience a heavy menstrual blood loss. This device has unfortunately not lived up to its early promise. While the volume of blood loss is reduced the frequency of bleeding is often greatly increased. There is also some concern about a greatly increased ectopic pregnancy risk among the small number of users who become pregnant.

Antigon (Denmark)

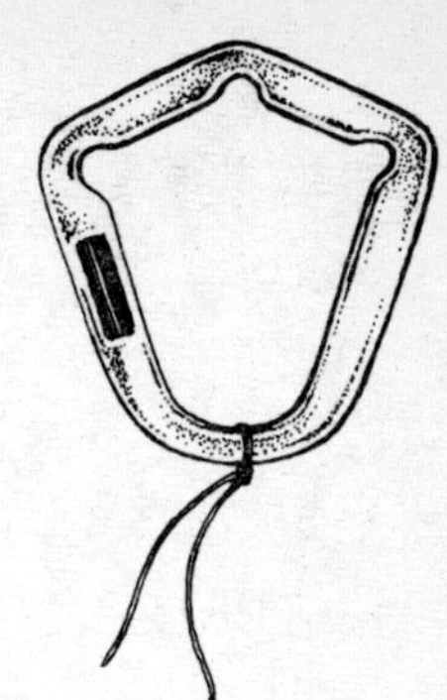

There are three versions of this IUD. The most recent (illustrated) has shown average pregnancy and expulsion risks but an abnormally high problem of increased bleeding and/or pain. The device is expected to pass through the cervical canal without reduction in size, and with a width of 26 mm at the widest point, considerable discomfort was reported at fitting. Very few doctors now fit this device.

Ota Ring (Japan)

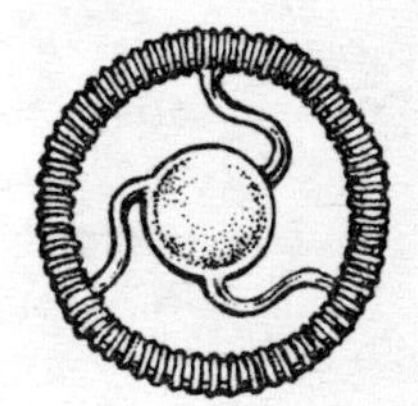

This is one of the earliest plastic devices and is worn by considerable numbers of Japanese women. It is not generally used in Western countries mainly because of the alleged discomfort at the time of fitting.

Levonorgestrel (Finland)

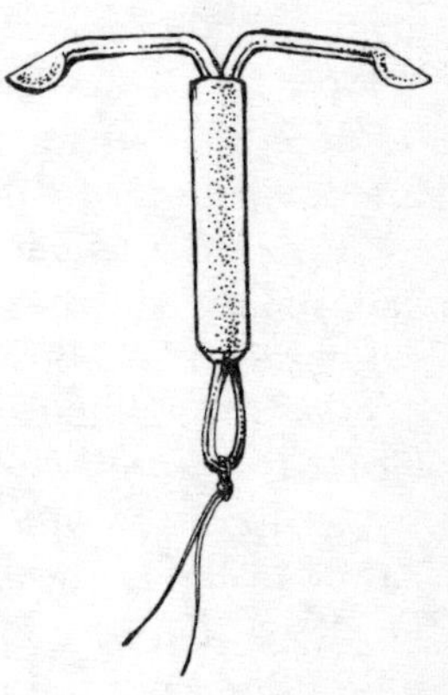

This hormone-releasing IUD is a successor to the Progestasert and is designed to release a progestogen directly into the uterus. It is hoped that this type of IUD will reduce the problem of bleeding still further and perhaps assist in the prevention of infection. This IUD is not yet generally available in sufficient numbers to provide an independent assessment of side effects.

GLOSSARY

Anaemia a deficiency in the number or quality of red blood cells, which depletes the oxygen carrying capacity of the blood

Anteverted tilted forwards

Anti-coagulant preventing clotting of the blood

Bimanual performed by both hands

Cervical canal the narrow passage running through the neck of the uterus or womb

Cervical erosion a disturbance of the mucus membrane surface cells at the junction of the cervical canal and the cervix itself

Cervix the neck of the uterus or womb

Contra-indication anything forbidding a particular method of treatment

Dysmenorrhoea painful periods

Ectopic pregnancy a pregnancy which occurs not in its proper place; i.e. outside the uterus

Endometrium the mucus membrane which is the inner lining of the uterine wall

External os the opening from the cervical canal into the vagina

Fallopian tube the oviduct. The fine tube leading from the ovary to the uterus or womb

Fibroid a fibrous, non-malignant (i.e. not cancerous) tumour of the uterus or womb

Fundus the farthest portion of a hollow organ

Implantation the embedding of the products of conception into the lining of the uterus or womb

Internal os the opening from the uterus or womb into the cervical canal

Macrophage a large scavenger cell

Menstruation the monthly periodic discharge of blood from the uterus or womb

Nulliparous not having borne children

Ovary the female reproductive gland containing ova or eggs

Ovum the egg or female sex cell

Parity the number of children a woman has borne

high parity having borne three or more children

low parity having borne one or two children

Parous having borne one or more children

Polyp a non-malignant (i.e. not cancerous) tumour which has a stalk

Post-coital after sexual intercourse

Post-partum the period of time just after childbirth

Retroverted tilted backwards

Speculum an instrument for bringing into view parts that are otherwise hidden

Sperm the male sex cell

Tenaculum an instrument for gripping and holding body tissue

Trimester a duration of three months. One-third of the length of a pregnancy

Uterine sound an elongated, cylindrical instrument used for exploring the uterine cavity

Uterine wall the muscular structure of the uterus or womb

Uterus the womb: the muscular organ which receives the fertilised egg and holds the developing foetus. Its muscular contractions expel the child at birth

Vagina the canal extending from the neck of the uterus (or womb) to the exterior

INDEX